W9-AXX-722

CANNABIS, ALCOHOL, AND THE
SOUTH AFRICAN STUDENT

Brian M. du Toit is a professor of Anthropology at the University of Florida, Gainesville, Florida 32611.

CANNABIS, ALCOHOL, AND THE SOUTH AFRICAN STUDENT

Adolescent Drug Use 1974-1985

by

Brian M. du Toit

Ohio University Center for International Studies
Monographs in International Studies

Africa Series Number 59
Athens, Ohio 1991

© Copyright 1991 by the
Center for International Studies

Printed in the United States of America
All rights reserved

The books in the Center for International Studies Monograph
Series are printed on acid-free paper ∞

Library of Congress Cataloging-in-Publication Data

du Toit, Brian M., 1935-
    Cannabis, alcohol, and the South African student :
adolescent drug use, 1974 – 1985
    p.   cm. – (Monographs in international studies.
Africa series; no. 59)
    Includes bibliographical references.
    ISBN 0-89680-166-7 (pbk.)
    1. High school students–South Africa–Drug use–Cross-
cultural studies. 2. High school students–South Africa–Alcohol
use–Cross-cultural studies. 3. High school students–South
Africa–Drug use–Longitudinal studies. 4. High school
students–South Africa–Alcohol use–Longitudinal studies. 5.
Drug abuse surveys–South Africa.
    I. Title. II. Series.
HV584. Y68D83   1991
362.29'21'0835–dc20   91–25451
                                                 CIP

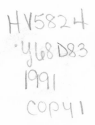

HV5824
·468 D83
1991
COPY1

CONTENTS

TABLES

CHART

ACKNOWLEDGEMENTS

A study such as this requires the support of a wide range of persons. Financial support from the Institute for Sociological and Demographic Research in the Human Sciences Research Council made this study possible. Regional inspectors, school principals, and classroom teachers associated with the twelve schools surveyed were not only supportive but also inquisitive and encouraging. Their wholehearted support despite a full and busy educational curriculum is greatly appreciated.

I thank the authorities who assisted in the formal arrangements. These include the Inspector of the Kwa Zulu Government Service (Blacks); the Executive Director of Education (Coloureds); the Chief Planner for the Director of Education (Indians); and the Chief Educational Planner for the Director of Education (Whites). In each case the regional inspector was involved as was the principal of each school. School principals were most hospitable and arranged for the space and time in a busy educational curriculum for senior students to complete the questionnaire. The students who participated were interested in the study, serious in their responses, and dedicated in their cooperation.

Much of the cross-cultural material referred to in the first chapter was collected by Lois Randolph. Her assistance is appreciated.

To all I say, thank you!

INTRODUCTION

When the 1974 study of drug use among South African students was published, I suggested that a similar one should be repeated among the same ethnic groups and in the same schools about 1984 (du Toit 1978:114). I anticipated that such a study would find changes in the patterns and attitudes concerning the drug use among Black, Indian, and Afrikaans students and that there would be a general increase in experimentation with other drugs. These questions form part of this inquiry.

As was the case in the previous report, I used proper names to indicate the four major "racial" or ethnic categories defined by law in South Africa. Thus, students attended segregated schools specifically designated as Black, Coloured, Indian, and White—these designations and spellings were retained.

The aim of this study was to survey cross-cultural use of drugs by adolescents and compare data collected a decade apart concerning attitudes and patterns of drug use among South African students. The focus was on *Cannabis sativa*, known locally as "dagga," and on alcohol. The advantage of the South African setting was the richness of linguistic and cultural traditions which permit the comparative study of groups and even subgroups. It is sad that these natural groups had been relegated to legal units which, by law, were allowed or denied mobility, actions, freedom and expression. For this reason I am extremely grateful to the students who were willing to respond honestly and openly to an extensive battery of questions.

A few remarks are in order regarding this book. The normal style of anthropologists to use the "ethnographic present" has been changed in this study. We speak here in the past tense. This is due in part to the time that has elapsed since the research was conducted and in part to the dramatic changes which have taken place in South African politics since 1990. These changes were actually introduced by the election of F. W. de Klerk as South

Africa's president. His bold and progressive initiatives resulted in the release of political prisoners, the suspension of executions, unbanning of political organizations (including the African National Congress, the Pan Africanist Congress, the South African Communist Party, and Umkhonto we Sizwe), and the allocation of finances specifically earmarked for "Black upliftment" to be administered by the Urban Foundation. More important, under de Klerk's leadership, the South African parliament repealed apartheid laws dealing with influx control, separate amenities, the Group Areas Act, and two Land Acts. These changes have been important for all minority groups but particularly so for Black South Africans. The result is that members of political minority groups will be free to move as they like and to reside where they prefer. Luckily changes in the educational policies also imply that we will not be able to repeat this study based on separate school facilities.

1

DRUG USE AMONG ADOLESCENTS:
A CROSS-CULTURAL PERSPECTIVE

Introduction

Adolescence is a time of extreme biological, psychological, and sociological change. It is an "Alice in Wonderland" kind of time when things can change so rapidly that to the adolescent the world seems very much out of focus, confusing, and switched about. To reconnoiter through such a world, Alice ate and drank substances to change herself. A similar response is not unusual among young people in many parts of the world today. Prior to 1965, drug patterns had remained the same for decades, and little attention was paid to adolescent drug-taking behavior because it was practically non-existent. Studies suggested that adolescents took drugs because of deviant personality formations caused by deprivation, anger, frustration, and rebellion. It was also suggested that they used drugs as therapeutic agents to alleviate psychological pain and stress caused by the maturation process.

In the 1960s licit and illicit drug use became a popular form of recreation among adolescents in the United States, crossing all ethnic, socio-economic, sex, and age barriers (Ungerleider and Andrysiak 1984). This form of experimentation also spread to other countries. Only by examining this phenomenon world-wide can we understand its profound implications. The use of drugs has become a common form of recreational activity pursued by an increasing number of young people in all parts of the world.

This chapter presents a cross-cultural examination of licit and illicit drug use among young people. It attempts to delineate some of the socio-cultural phenomena involved and the particular demographic characteristics of the sample populations. We may not be able to abolish drug use among young people, but through

1

definition and analysis we can seek to better understand the phenomenon. Only in this way can we make intelligent policy decisions regarding education, therapy, and legislative control of both licit and illicit drugs.

United States of America

The "drug scene" in America changed greatly from the period prior to the 1960s to the mid-1980s (Ungerleider and Andrysiak 1984). Not only are students experimenting with a myriad of both licit and illicit drugs, they are also using these drugs together to obtain a synergistic effect. Etiology has variously been attributed to several psycho-social correlates (Brawcht 1973; Wechsler and Thum 1973; Kaplan and Pokorny 1978; Jessor and Jessor 1977; McLaughlin et al. 1985), to parental and peer use (Igra and Moos 1979; Britt and Campbell 1977; Braucht 1980; Margulies et al. 1977; Downs 1987; Dishion and Loeber 1985; Rooney 1983; Alexander and Campbell 1966; and Kandel 1973), and to stages of adolescent involvement in drug use (Kandel 1975).

Some studies (Wechsler and McFadden 1976; Kandel, Single, and Kessler 1976; Downs 1987) suggest that gender differences of those most frequently using drugs are disappearing. The researchers observe that "adolescent females have a normative structure that is as positive toward alcohol as that of adolescent males" (Downs 1987:174). Since it is now as acceptable for adolescent females to participate in drug-taking behavior, females are consuming as many drugs as males.

A majority of the studies on licit and illicit drug use among adolescents in the U.S. has concentrated on the role of peers and parents. Most of these studies postulate that peer and parental alcohol use are primary predictors of adolescent drug-taking activity. It is not clear, however, whether adolescents use drugs and then seek out as friends others who use drugs or whether friends influence one another to use drugs. The role of the relationship of parental use as an influence on adolescent drug use is also unclear. Does it demonstrate effects of modeling, of genetic predisposition, or a combination of both? Researchers are struggling with these questions, and as yet have found no definitive answer. To show trends in drug use in the United States, this discussion concentrates on four regional studies

2

(Blackford 1977; du Toit and Suggs 1985; Kandel et al. 1976; Murray et al. 1987) and a national study encompassing the nine years from 1976 to 1984 (Johnston and O'Malley 1986; Johnston, Bachman and O'Malley 1984).

Blackford (1977) studied drug use among students in San Mateo County, California from 1968 to 1977. The sample ranged in size from 18,774 to 31,251 people. The study revealed that students drinking alcoholic beverages in grades nine to twelve increased from 65.4 percent to 88 percent in the years 1968-1977. Those using cannabis increased from 31.9 percent to 57.5 percent in the years 1968-1977. Rates of increase were generally higher among females than males. Among females, twice as many used cannabis in 1977 as in 1968.

Kandel et al. (1976) undertook a two-wave panel survey in a representative sample of New York secondary school students in the fall of 1971 and the spring of 1972. Using a stratified sample of eighteen high schools, they collected structured, self-administered questionnaires from 8,206 adolescents. Their findings suggest that the majority of adolescents (82 percent) had drunk beer or wine, smoked cigarettes (72 percent), or used hard liquor (65 percent). Over one-third (35 percent) had used one or more illegal drugs, the most frequent being marijuana (29 percent) and hashish (21 percent). A further finding was that although a smaller proportion used marijuana than hard liquor, those who tried marijuana were more likely to become heavy, current, and regular users than those who tried hard liquor. An additional finding of interest was that there were stages in adolescent drug use. According to these researchers, the legal drugs including beer, wine, hard liquor, and cigarettes seem to be necessary inter-mediaries between nonuse and marijuana use. While 27 percent of the high school students in this sample who smoked and drank progressed to marijuana within a five-to-six month follow-up period, only 2 percent of those who had not used any legal substance did so (Kandel 1975).

In 1983 du Toit conducted a survey on drug use among high school students in a county in the state of Florida. The focus of the study was on attitudes about and patterns of use of a variety of drugs but especially cannabis and alcohol. These findings have been reported respectively in du Toit and Suggs (1985) and Suggs and du Toit (1985). Questionnaires were administered and were

3

completed by 72 percent of ninth graders and 61 percent of twelfth graders from a total sample size of 3,140. The results showed that males were more likely than females to use both cannabis and alcohol. Regular users were likely also to have used both drugs prior to high school. Eighty-four percent of the males and 80 percent of the females had used alcohol at least once or twice; 40 percent of the males and 26 percent of the females had used it twenty times or more. Fifty-two percent of the males and 41 percent of the females had used marijuana at least once or twice; 17 percent of the males and 11 percent of the females had used it twenty times or more.

In the Minneapolis and St. Paul metropolitan area, 4,599 seventh grade students were surveyed between October and November of 1983 (Murray et al. 1987). Tobacco was used by 11.1 percent of the twelve-year-olds and 15.6 of the thirteen-year-olds. More females (13.3 percent) than males smoked tobacco. Of the twelve-year-olds, 27.5 percent reported use of alcohol while 9.9 percent described themselves as heavy drinkers. More males (12.4 and 30.9) drank alcohol than females (9.0 and 12.4). Students were asked if they used marijuana, and 5.4 percent of the twelve-year-olds and 10.1 percent of the thirteen-year-olds answered in the affirmative. Again, more males (8.0 percent) than females (5.0 percent) said they used marijuana. Using multivariate analysis, the researchers reported some important findings. Data showed that female seventh graders were equal to males in their susceptibility to drug use. The study found that black and white students had the same prevalence of monthly use of tobacco, alcohol, and marijuana. Students who lived in female headed households were 1.6 times more likely to have smoked marijuana during the previous month. Also, children whose mothers held white-collar jobs were more likely to drink and use marijuana.

Johnston and O'Malley (1986) and Johnston, O'Malley, and Bachman (1984) in their analysis of trends nationwide between 1976 and 1984 noted that reasons for using drugs have shown only a modest degree of change while prevalence rates for some drugs have changed substantially. Alcohol and marijuana were the drugs of choice for the majority of young people in the United States. The population sample used in their study consisted of all seniors enrolled in public and private high schools in the USA. Representative samples of from 16,000 to 19,000 students were

4

drawn from 130 schools. The student response rate ranged from 77 percent to 84 percent. Confidentiality was assured to all respondents. In the class of 1984, 86 percent of the students reported using alcohol in the previous twelve months; 40 percent reported using marijuana or hashish. It is interesting to note that while marijuana usage was actually down 4.5 percent from 1976, use of cocaine almost doubled from 6 percent in 1976 to 11.6 percent in 1984. Recreational reasons for drug taking were preponderant over therapeutic or psychological reasons. Sixty-five percent of the students reported taking drugs "to have a good time with my friends." This reason is not to be confused with peer pressure since only 13 percent reported taking drugs "to fit in with a group I like." Fifty-four percent wanted to "experiment and see what it's like" and 49 percent "to feel good or get high." Only 22 percent took drugs to "get away from my problems." Seventy-eight percent used cocaine "to experiment, see what its like," while only 41 percent used alcohol for this reason. Conversely, 73 percent used alcohol to "have a good time with my friends," while only 50 percent used cocaine for this reason. Sixty-three percent of the marijuana users cited experimentation while 65 percent said using facilitated "having a good time with my friends."

When it treated drug use among adolescents at all, the literature prior to the 1970s suggested that drugs were used by troubled or deviant teenagers who sought an escape from anger or frustration, a way to get away from their problems. In the late 1980s this was no longer the case. The vast majority of teenagers then cited recreational reasons for using drugs. Only a small minority said they used drugs "because of anger and frustration" (18 percent) or "to get away from problems or troubles" (21 percent). Perhaps it is difficult for adults brought up thinking of drugs as substances used by deviant or psychologically disturbed adolescents to understand the use of drugs as one of many recreational pursuits open to young people who have increasing amounts of money and leisure time.

Pinto (1973) described substance abuse among Native American youth as "a major national scandal." From 1975 to 1981 there had been increasing use of both licit and illicit drugs among adolescents living on reservations. Beauvais, Oetting, and Edwards (1985) issued anonymous surveys on drug use to seventh through twelfth grade students attending Indian reservation schools.

During the year 1980-1981, using a sample of 2,159 students, the researchers found that one-fourth of the students had been drunk at least once during the two months prior to the survey. Eighty-nine percent of Indian youth had tried alcohol and 74.2 percent had tried marijuana. It was estimated that about 50 percent of Indian young people were at risk through their drug and alcohol use.

Perspectives concerning why alcohol and drug use were so prevalent on reservations suggest that Indian adolescent attitudes about drinking were influenced by a norm of approval and strong tolerance of the activity in the communities (Cockerham 1975; 1977; Swanson et al. 1971; Topper 1974) and permissive child rearing practices (Swanson 1971). Several studies implied that components of Native American culture, or rather the disruption of their traditional values and culture, may explain the high rate of alcohol and drug use (May 1982; Medicine 1982; Weibel-Orlando 1984). Economically Native Americans are one of the most impoverished groups in American society and have a low educational level. Prejudice against them is rampant and they have very little political power. Health care is extremely poor. In view of these circumstances, it is not surprising to find that suicide rates (Dizmang et al. 1974) and juvenile offenses (Jensen et al. 1977) were well above the national average.

Native American youth began their use of drugs at an earlier age than their white counterparts. A study of drug use among fourth to sixth graders (Oetting and Goldstein 1978) showed that 30 percent of the sample drank beer, 6.8 percent used inhalants, and 2.5 percent had tried "pills." The researchers suggest that three major factors influence drug use: wide use of drugs within the community, few negative sanctions, and peer and sibling encouragement.

Some studies (Weibel 1982) suggest that the majority of urban Indians living off the reservation do not have as great a problem with substance abuse as those living on the reservation, perhaps because they have a "stake" in American society (Ferguson 1968). Murray et al. sum up the problem of adolescent drug use among Native American youth as follows:

> Several reasons have been suggested for greater drug use among Native American adolescents. They may

face rejection based on their race. They often grow up in and face a life of poverty. There are major conflicts between traditional Indian values and contemporary American values. Those who remain on the reservation face limited employment and recreational opportunities. Those who leave the reservation may face sudden cultural disruption and lose the strong family support systems which have been an important part of traditional Indian life. Growing up as a Native American adolescent has been described as a difficult and stressful experience, and drug use may be a frequent response (1987:371).

It is obvious from the literature that use of both licit and illicit drugs for recreational reasons is endorsed by many of the youth in the USA. A cross-cultural review of the literature will suggest whether this is simply a trend in an affluent Western country with lots of money and leisure time or whether it is endorsed by young people worldwide.

Canada

Using large proportionate samples of students in grades seven, nine, eleven, and thirteen between 1968 and 1974, Smart et al. (1979) found that the percentage of drinkers increased from 46.3 percent in 1968 to 72.9 percent in 1974. Though the percentage of drinkers between 1977 and 1979 did not increase (76.3 percent and 76.9 percent), the percentage of those with drug-related problems did increase. Between 1968 and 1979 the greatest differences were measured among females. Drinking and heavy drinking were most common, however, among males, older students, those who were doing poorly in school, and those with solid, middle class socio-economic backgrounds. From 1968 to 1970 cannabis use increased 11.6 percent. From 1970 to 1979 drug use increased 13.4 percent. Increases were larger among females than males. In 1979 31.7 percent of Canada's youth reported some use of cannabis. Overall, cannabis use was more common among males, students with lower grades, and those from middle-class socio-economic backgrounds. Eleventh-grade students

7

reported greater prevalence than thirteenth-grade students (Smart and Murray 1981).

Australia

Studies pertaining to the use of licit and illicit drugs have been conducted in New South Wales since 1971. Champion et al. (1978) studied 500 tenth grade students in 1977 and compared usage levels with 1971 and 1973 figures reported by Bell et al. (1975). In 1977 the percentage of students reporting that all or some of their friends used cannabis climbed from 30 percent to 62 percent. Students showed a reduced perception of the dangers of both alcohol and cannabis.

The most recent survey was in *Social Science Data Archives*, 1983. A sample of 4,165 students aged from twelve to seventeen were surveyed using questionnaires resembling those used by Bachman and Johnston (1978). At this time, alcohol was the most common drug problem. There were few differences in consumption patterns between males and females. At age twelve, 70 percent of the males and 60 percent of the females were familiar with alcohol. About 14 percent of sixteen-year-old boys and 12 percent of sixteen-year-old girls drink alcohol daily. By age sixteen, 90 percent of the students reported having drunk alcohol. About 53 percent of the boys and 39 percent of the girls stated that they drank five or more drinks on occasions when they drink. About half of the students claim to have drunk to the point of being sick, and 20 percent of the students reported passing out. The study showed that "there exists a significant group of adolescent drinkers whose purpose in drinking alcohol is to get drunk" (Homel and Flaherty 1986:205).

Scandinavia

Denmark. In Denmark a study of adolescent drug use was done between 1960 and 1974 (Sindballe 1978). Comparative data was collected using a survey administered to 1,381 high school students in 1963 and administering the identical survey to two separate groups of 3,428 twelve to twenty-year-olds and 2,009 twelve to eighteen-year-olds. These data show that average annual consumption of alcohol doubled between 1960 and 1974.

Frequency of drinking was also shown to increase (Smart and Murray 1981).

Finland. In Finland a series of studies conducted in 1960 and again in 1973 and three consecutive studies in 1977, 1978, and 1979 showed that consumption of alcohol more than tripled from 1960 to 1974. The percentage of boys and girls who used alcohol in 1979 was the same. The number of students using alcohol daily declined between 1973 and 1979 (Ahlstrom-Laakso 1979).

Norway. Yearly studies were conducted in Oslo on sample sizes ranging from 1,027 in 1969 to 739 in 1979 (Irgens-Jensen 1979). Alcohol use remained stable but cannabis use fluctuated, with an increase from 5.3 percent in 1968 to 18.8 percent in 1972, a drop to 16.5 percent in 1976 to a further rise to 22.5 percent in 1979. Differences in cannabis use by sex declined. In 1975 and 1976 equal numbers of males and females used cannabis. A second Norwegian study using three surveys (Brun-Gulbrandsen 1978) showed that alcohol use increased from 69 percent in 1956 to 93 percent in 1973.

Sweden. In 1956, 1961, and 1967, questionnaires were administered to a sample of 1,435 students, who showed significant increases in the consumption and regular use of alcohol. The number of adults in student families who did not drink decreased from 42 percent to 31 percent. Attitudes toward alcohol were much more liberal (Hofsten 1969). In a second study several surveys were conducted between 1947 and 1976. In one survey with a sample size ranging from 8,300 to 13,400, students replied to questionnaires distributed over a six year period from 1971-1976. Increases in alcohol consumption were recorded for each year. Age of first use decreased and quantities consumed per occasion increased.

France

Alcoholism is one of the foremost public-health problems in France, yet only three studies (Davidson 1973, 1974; IREB 1976) of adolescent drug use have been carried out (Kandel et al. 1981). Kandel (1981) citing the growing concern over drug use in many

9

countries and the too few epidemiological cross-cultural data available, decided to survey adolescents in France and Israel in order to make a comparative analysis. Using a survey conducted in 1977, the French sample included 499 French adolescents between fourteen and eighteen years old from Paris and surrounding suburbs. Structured interview schedules were administered to households. Data pertained to lifetime and current prevalences and sociodemographic correlates of patterns of use. Only 23 percent of French youth had tried marijuana but 82 percent reported using tobacco. Eighty percent had drunk beer, 79 percent wine, and 75 percent hard liquor. Almost equal numbers of males and females drank alcohol, including 81 percent of the males and 77 percent of the females for wine and 79 percent of the males and 70 percent of the females for hard liquor. Twenty-six percent of the males and 18 percent of the females reported smoking marijuana. Seventy-five percent had sampled alcohol by age fourteen. By age eighteen 91 percent had drunk hard liquor. Religiosity seems to be correlated with drinking practices in France. Only 50 percent of those attending church more than once a month had tried hard liquor as compared with 77 percent of those who were nonreligious. There was no correlation between licit and illicit drug use and socioeconomic indicators such as father's occupation.

Israel

Kandel et al. (1981) also studied drug use among Israeli adolescents. His population sample consisted of 609 Israeli youth between the ages of fourteen and eighteen. All of the subjects resided in major urban centers. Ritualistic and nonritualistic uses of wine were distinguished. Again, data pertained to lifetime and current prevalences and sociodemographic indicators. The lifetime prevalence of use of illegal drugs was exceedingly small. Only 3 percent of Israeli youth reported having ever used marijuana. No Israeli youth reported ever having used LSD, amphetamines, or heroin. In the last thirty days before the questionnaire was administered, only 27 percent of Israeli youth reported drinking beer or wine, and only 22 percent reported using hard liquor. Only 4 percent reported drinking hard liquor more than ten times in their lives. At eighteen years old, only 64 percent had sampled hard liquor; 38 percent reported having tasted hard liquor by age fourteen. There was a considerable difference between male and female usage. While 79 percent, 72 percent, and 61 percent of the males had respectively tried beer, wine, and hard liquor, only 62 percent, 55 percent and 44 percent of the females had drunk beer, wine, or liquor. Religiosity appeared to be an insignificant deterrent. Seventy-three percent of nonreligious youth reported drinking beer as compared with 61 percent of religious youth. For wine the percentages were 58 and 53. The nonreligious sample had tried hard liquor less than the religious sample (56 percent). There was no consistent relationship between adolescent drug use and socioeconomic correlates.

South America

Mexico. One short-term study of drug use among adolescents in Mexico (Castro 1980) was reported by Smart and Murray (1981). Data pertained to alcohol use only and was based on a national sample of students between fourteen and eighteen years old. Between 1976 and 1978, 3.5 times as many students reported drinking alcohol, and the rate of increase was greater among females than males.

Medina-Mora et al. (1981) reported that several surveys of drug use among Mexican students had been done (Lafarga 1972; Cabildo et al. 1972; Carranza-Acevedo et al. 1972; De la Fuenti 1972; Wellishch and Hays 1974; Castro and Chao 1976). Using the questionnaire developed by Smart (1980) Medina-Mora et al. (1981) chose as a sample twelve groups of students from seven high-risk schools. The population included both urban and rural students. Both sexes were equally represented. The researchers administered two tests to validate the original data. In the first test, 42.9 percent of the subjects reported having used alcohol. In the second test, 41.1 percent said they had used alcohol. On the first test, 5.1 percent reported using cannabis and on the second test, 4.8 percent reported usage.

Chile. Surveys conducted between 1968 and 1970 (Gomberoff et al. 1972) reported a 6.96 percent prevalence rate of cannabis use among 734 high school students in Chile. It was proposed in this study that students who used alcohol and whose parents used

11

alcohol were more apt to use cannabis. In another Chilean study (Urzua et al. 1982), a questionnaire was administered to 1,240 high school students in Santiago. There were an equal number of males and females. The majority (76.6 percent) were between fourteen and seventeen years of age. Alcohol was used by 70.5 percent of the subjects and cannabis by 7.3 percent. Tobacco was used by 56.3 percent of the students. Frequent use of alcohol (taking alcoholic beverages one or more times a week) was reported by 14.5 percent of the students, and 32 percent reported intoxication. Alcohol was usually imbibed at parties or social gatherings (39 percent). Hard liquor was used more than beer or wine. Seventeen percent of the students had tried cannabis and 7.3 percent continued using it. The main reason given for using cannabis was curiosity (55.6 percent). Males used alcohol more frequently than female students and more often became intoxicated. The use of cannabis was also more frequent among males than females. Occasional use of alcohol was almost equal for males and females (343 males and 349 females), but occasional use of cannabis was more frequent among males (fifty-five males and eleven females). There was a steady increase in the use of drugs between the first and third year of high school, with a slight decrease in the fourth year. Most of the frequent users were male students from one of the higher income groups. The majority of frequent users also lived with both parents (68.7 percent for alcohol and 58.3 percent for cannabis). Fathers tended to be professionals and mothers housewives, although there was a higher percentage of professional mothers of students in the group of frequent users. Most frequent users reported antipathy on the part of parents toward drug use, with more conflicts resulting. Frequent users also showed some degree of social maladjustment.

Africa

Zambia. Nyambe (1979) as reported by Haworth (1982) conducted a study on the use of cannabis by young people in Zambia before and after independence in 1964. He suggested that there was a great increase in cannabis smoking after independence, with 50,000 juveniles appearing before courts for cannabis smoking between 1964 and 1978. Haworth (1982) disputes Nyambe's claims and says they cannot be substantiated by police records. He did his own study of secondary schools in Zambia. Using a sample size of 336 students from five secondary schools, he found that 58 percent of the males and 57 percent of the females had consumed alcohol. Thirty-two percent of the males and 26 percent of the females had taken drugs at some time; 5.6 percent of the students reported drinking alcohol at least once a week while, 3.4 percent reported using cannabis at least once a week. Cannabis was used more frequently by males, and there was an increase in usage with age from 6 percent at twelve to fourteen years of age to 47 percent at nineteen years of age or more. Ten percent of the females in the age group fifteen to sixteen years used cannabis. Males were more likely to smoke cannabis and females to take drugs such as tranquilizers.

Nigeria. Anumonya (1980) conducted a study of secondary schools in Lagos. The sample of 2,846 pupils was drawn from seventeen secondary schools. Students' ages ranged from eleven to twenty years, and there was an equal distribution of males and females. Data were based on responses to questionnaires. There was a fairly even distribution of both alcohol and cannabis use among males and females. Surprisingly, slightly more females (21.1 percent) than males (20.7 percent) used alcohol, and more males (2.9 percent) than females (2.1 percent) used cannabis.

Between 1977 and 1979, 1,500 secondary school students in Bendel State, Nigeria, were interviewed (Nevadomsky 1981). Fifty-five percent of the students had used alcohol, with more males (72 percent) than females (45 percent) responding in the affirmative. More females (46 percent) than males admitted using tranquilizers. Ten percent of the student population had tried marijuana, although more than twice as many males (15 percent) as females (six percent) use the drug. According to other studies done in Nigeria (Nevadomsky 1981:16), 49 percent of the students in Nigeria used drugs out of curiosity. Thirty-eight percent used them because friends did, and 37 percent cited feeling good and enjoying social occasions. Only 25 percent used them for therapeutic or psychological reasons—to stay calm or avoid anxiety. Of drugs currently used, alcohol was the more prevalent, among 19 percent of the sample of students in Bendel State. Only six percent were then using marijuana. Nevadomsky concluded that

13

on the whole, secondary school students disapprove of most forms of drug use among their peers and very few of them actually use drugs regularly . . . The evidence is therefore convincing that the stresses of secondary school adolescence, as they exist in the Bendel State of Nigerian society, have not resulted in wide scale drug abuse. (1981:18)

Students in the Nigerian towns of Warri and Effurun also were interviewed (Nevadomsky 1982). Data was collected on 260 males and 224 females using a questionnaire modeled on the one given to students in previous drug research projects conducted in Africa by du Toit (1978). Average age of students in the sample was 27.5 years for males and 16.8 years for females. No significant association was found between drug use and the social and demographic characteristics of the students. The majority of students (60 percent) professed some religious affiliation while 36 percent described themselves as very religious. Thirty percent of the students' fathers were businessmen, 27 percent unskilled workers, 17 percent civil servants, and 26 percent professionals. Eighty-two percent of the students said they were on good terms with their parents and another 14 percent said they got along all right. Only 4 percent had problems with parents. Fifty percent of the students belonged to social clubs. About two-thirds of the students, both male and female, had some experience with alcohol. Twice as many males (37 percent) as females (16 percent) smoked cigarettes, while more females (19.2 percent) than males (15 percent) used tranquilizers. More males (7.7 percent) than females (5.8 percent) used cannabis. Nearly three-quarters of the students who used drugs frequently were multiple drug users. A typical pattern was spirits, beer, and tobacco. No relationship between age and initial exposure could be determined. Sixty-three percent of the males and 58 percent of the females said they used cannabis outside of school. The majority of students thought their parents would disapprove of drug use, and parental use of drugs appeared limited. The main reason given for not using drugs was the risk of being damaged mentally and physically. The main reason cited for using drugs was to be social and get along with friends. The majority of students (83 percent) felt that those who used drugs were not much different from those who did not.

Though drugs are readily available in Nigeria from shops and supermarkets with no age restrictions, there is no widespread use of drugs among Nigeria's secondary school students. What use there is appears to be "normal" rather than "pathological." The majority of students who do use drugs, use them to have a good time and get along with friends (Nevadomsky 1982:31).

Summary

A review of research reports presents us with a number of interesting conclusions. As can be expected in cultures where alcohol use is sanctioned while cannabis and most other drugs are illegal, alcohol use is consistently higher among students. A variety of studies of student groups in the United States consistently found frequencies of 80 percent or more of the sample to have used alcohol. The figure for cannabis ranged from a low of about 30 percent to a high of almost 75 percent on an Indian Reservation. While most researchers discount socio-economic, familial, and related demographic factors as being causal, conditions among reservation residents do require special attention to these factors (see Levy and Kunitz 1974; du Toit 1964).

Turning to international patterns of use, we are faced with a major problem, namely what is drug use? Most studies use as criterion the question of whether a person had "ever used" a particular substance. Some studies tend to differentiate between experimentation and use. The highest figures for alcohol use by adolescents was found in Australia and Norway, both 90 percent and above. Smart and Murray, who saw a correlation between alcohol and cannabis use, concluded that "the rates of alcohol use have reached a peak in many countries which cannot be easily exceeded (80 to 90 percent) because the remaining abstainers have strong religious beliefs or illnesses which prohibit drinking" (1981:8). In Norway cannabis use was up to 22.5 percent in 1979, and in Australia 62.0 percent of the adolescents reported it.

Israel is well documented as having a low incidence of cannabis use, but figures for Mexico are suspect. There is a pattern emerging in Africa in which students give a negative evaluation to drug use. We would differentiate between students and nonstudents. As can be expected, males are generally more willing to experiment, and show higher figures for use whether it is alcohol in Nigeria, cannabis in France, or both drugs in the American South. What is needed is a greater uniformity in testing devices or questionnaires and also greater uniformity in reporting. This would maximize comparability of research findings and plotting of trends.

One word of caution. It is incumbent upon a researcher to indicate whether the subjects were students or just adolescents, including age mates who had left school. Readers should take note that frequently there is a higher rate of use among those who have dropped out of school or taken a job. It can be proposed also that the highest rate of drug use might be before twelfth grade. The higher students go in the academic ladder the more serious they become. In some situations, however, this is balanced by greater freedom and greater availability of mind-altering substances.

2

THE SOUTH AFRICAN DRUG STUDY
1974-1985

Introduction

While American students were heartily experimenting with uppers and downers, their white South African counterparts were cautiously breaking the cannabis barrier. While LSD and similar mind altering substances were common elements for the more daring student in American high schools, their agemates in South Africa hardly had heard about these drugs. While state legislatures and the highest office in the U.S. talked of legalizing the use of "pot," *Cannabis sativa* in South Africa was classified with heroin, opium, and LSD as "Prohibited Dependence-producing Drugs."

The reasons for these differences are complex and are presented in greater detail in a number of publications listed in the bibliography. It would be sufficient at this stage merely to suggest the more obvious ones.

Background

When Europeans under the Dutch East Indies Company settled at the Cape in 1652, cannabis already was smoked by indigenous groups, including Khoikhoi, San, and Bantu speakers. For the next three centuries, Whites associated this drug primarily with the traditional Black population and secondly with a lower socioeconomic lifestyle. The latter lifestyle implied an absence or loss of Christian values, degradation, and of course, escapism in the form of mind altering experiences.

There existed, however, two other major population groups, namely Indians and Coloureds. In 1860 the *Truro* sailed from Madras with Indian migrant laborers who were supposed to work

17

on a temporary basis in the Natal sugar plantations. These new arrivals brought with them a tradition of cannabis use. Soon after arrival they had established supply networks from the local Zulu and started their own gardens. In time they became permanent residents of South Africa and today constitute the largest group of Indians outside the Indian subcontinent and Sri Lanka. The Coloureds are the offspring of members of the previously mentioned groups as well as other ethnic groups such as the Malays who originally served as slaves to the early Dutch settlers.

As suggested, the Black and Indian population groups had long-standing traditions of cannabis use. These traditions had ritual and religious overtones and frequently had medicinal and curative contexts. Due partly to the association of cannabis with the laboring color caste, i.e., Black, and partly to the negative connotation of altered states of consciousness, Whites frowned on the use of drugs and abhorred the smoking of cannabis. In time the people who were classified as Coloured may have initiated the smoking of cannabis due in part to association with members of the lower color castes and in part to their frustrating marginal situation.

By the early 1970s it was not unusual for young South Africans, of whatever ethnic classification, to smoke cannabis at parties. Many of these youths smoked the drug on a regular basis and the believed association between ethnic group and/or lower socioeconomic class with cannabis use was rapidly disappearing.

South Africa's Ethnic Groups

Before outlining the research which underlies this study and discussing the research sample, it would be useful to clarify in some greater detail the position of the major ethnic groups. For reasons of comparison and because of differing cultural traditions, we will compare the indigenous Black with White settlers, Indian migrants, and the mestizo Coloured population.

Aboriginal Black Settlers. As far as we know today, the first people to occupy the southern part of Africa were hunters and gatherers and perhaps also herders. These groups, who were occupying the Cape when the Portuguese first rounded the southern tip of Africa, have gained a place in literature known as the "Bushmen" and "Hottentot." These terms of reference have, however, created a great deal of confusion.

The Europeans tended to lump together all yellow-skinned, hunting-and-gathering peoples whose language was characterized by "clicks." These people were called "Bushmen" after the early reference of Bosjesmans assigned by the Dutch settlers to the little people who would appear, as if out of nowhere, from behind a shrub or bush. They were differentiated from the yellow-skinned people, taller in stature, who also employed "clicks" in their language but who were cattle and sheep herders. The latter were called "Hottentot," possibly due to the stammering sound effected by their language. In time anthropological literature contained descriptions of yellow-skinned people who employed various "clicks" in their language. They could be differentiated on the following bases:

1. Culturally, by the fact of herding versus hunting and gathering
2. Linguistically, by the kind of language they employed
3. Physically, by stature and a few other minor traits

Among themselves the aboriginal settlers of the Cape had differentiated between the "Khoina" or "men of men" as the herders referred to themselves, and the "sana" referring to all yellow-skinned hunters and gatherers. Today it has become accepted—partly because a derogatory note is now attached to the term "Hottentot"—to refer to all these peoples as the Khoisan or to differentiate between the Khoikhoi and the San. There is a growing insistence that when physical descriptions or names are used, these be based on physical criteria only. Linguistic classifications should be based on linguistic criteria. One of the persons who has made this insistence on the clearest linguistic grounds is Westphal (1963 and 1971), who was rewriting the linguistic prehistory of southern Africa. However, Elphick (1977) confused the dichotomy by speaking about the Khoikhoi and the hunters.

In addition to the Khoisan groups, there existed also a few groups of Negro hunters who were marked by an extremely simple material culture. Some of these spoke a Khoikhoi language (Nama), and they are together referred to as the "Dama,"

"Damara," or "Bergdama." There will be an occasional reference to them in our discussion of cannabis use.

The first people which the Portuguese met when they rounded the Cape in 1487 were yellow-skinned herders. They were not settled villagers but seemed to migrate in response to available grazing and water supplies and build temporary camps. According to the diary and description of Jan van Riebeeck, the first Dutch commander at the Cape, they met small groups of Khoikhoi who made a living from hunting, fishing, and collecting along the seashore. These people became known as the Strandloopers (literally "Beach Walkers").

The first Portuguese observers were confused by various preparations which were eaten or drunk (and did not contain cannabis), preparations which were smoked in various mixtures (which included cannabis), and products which were smelled and inhaled (which might have included cannabis but were usually restricted to roots such as the gannabossie, the Ganna shrub). Jan van Riebeeck, six years after arriving at the Cape, reported on the *daccha*, which the herders ate in the form of a dry powder. It is almost certain that this was either gannabossie or more likely *Leonotis leonurus*. Its leaves were also frequently smoked—either alone or mixed with tobacco.

Ten Rhyne's (1968) mention of datura is of particular interest since a number of species are found in southern Africa. Whites, no doubt affected by early Khoikhoi cultural influences, used to smoke *Datura stramonium* for asthma and bronchitis (Watt and Breyer-Brandwijk 1932:166) while the Tsonga used *Datura fastuosa* in ordeals and also in the puberty initiation for young girls (Johnston 1977). Whether there was a terminological confusion between datura and dagga is not clear, but we do know that among others the leaf of the *Cineraria aspera* today is smoked by some southern Bantu speakers, and it is said to be as intoxicating as cannabis.

It will be noticed that in almost all cases thus far we may be dealing with *Leonotis leonurus* and other shrubs and not with *Cannabis sativa*, though all references are to dagga. We know that dagga, referring specifically to cannabis, was grown domestically, for Mentzel, writing in 1785, explains that white settlers who employed Khoikhoi paid them with "a few head of cattle, a little tobacco, dagga, some knives, [and] glass beads" (1944:85). Latrobe, in fact, was so incensed at this use of dacha, as he referred to "a species of wild hemp (cicuta)," that he proposed the first penal code against its use and distribution—a penalty fully as severe as that which exists today.

> It is necessary, therefore, that most determined resistance should be made against this destructive propensity, and by a rule established in our settlements, the use of dacha is to be entirely abandoned. Whoever is smoking it, is excluded: but a seducer of others to the abominable practice, expelled. (1969:334)

He was disturbed that those very persons who complain about the custom among the Khoikhoi "should encourage the growth of it in their grounds, and sell it to the Hottentots."

In addition to the use of dagga at this time, we also find reference to the use of kanna among the Khoikhoi and the San. Kanna was a root which was greatly valued as it was burned and the smoke inhaled (Kolb 1968:210-12). Arbousset and Daumas, writing of a San community they visited in the Free State, said that "the old mamma took from her neck a bit of some narcotic root, lit it at the fire; and bringing it near her nose, snuffed in the smoke" (1846:251). This seems to have been a common practice for Stow also describes it (1905:53).

In addition it seems that the leaves of the ganna bush were "also dried and powdered, and used both for chewing and smoking. When mixed with dacha it was very intoxicating" (Stow 1905:53). In a different source, Lichtenstein (1928:154) identifies it as *Salsola aphylla* and *Salicornia fruticosa* and as being used by indigenous peoples and white settlers. We are told that kanna, canna, or ganna could be identified as "several species of Salsola" which were chewed in much the same way "as the natives of India use betel or areca" (Schapera and Farrington 1933, footnote pages 264-65). It was thus another of a group of stimulants used by the Khoisan peoples.

While so many of the early writers used the term "dagga" without clearly identifying it, we would suggest that all along they might have been observing the use of *Cannabis sativa* along with other herbs and roots. Among the latter we must certainly include different species of leonotis and salsola. The question remains whether the smoking of cannabis was introduced by the relatively late arrival of the Negroid migrants or whether it had been present among hunters and herders prior to the arrival of the Negroid cultivators. One thing can be accepted without doubt: smoking long preceded the arrival of Whites in southern Africa. It is thus difficult to understand on what basis Raven-Hart states that the indigenous "wild dagga" was chewed, since "the idea of smoking anything came in with the Dutch" (1971:507).

During their southward migration the Bantu-speaking Negroids spread their gardens and claimed as pastures most of the eastern and northern parts of southern Africa. Our ethno-historical discussion will start in the south because documents which are readily available recount early meetings first on the eastern frontier and later further north and east.

As White settlers and explorers moved eastward from the founding settlement, later known as Cape Town, they met the Xhosa, Fingo and other southern Nguni people. In 1807, Alberti reported that among the Xhosa smoking was practiced by men and women (as is still the case) and both tobacco and cannabis were valued (Alberti 1968:25). Andrew Smith, who gained a very thorough knowledge of the Nguni people, stated that "Dakka has from time immemorial been known to the Caffers. They are very partial to smoking it. Those that can procure both tobacco and dakka snuff the former and smoke the latter. They smoke it through water" (1939:312). Much the same description is given by Baines (1964:213). Andrew Smith also mentions the smoking of cannabis among the Baralong and Bathlapin—both subgroups of the Tswana. The smoking of hemp by the Bechuana, another Tswana group, is also mentioned by Conder (1887:82). Baines gives a full description of the water pipe and also presents a drawing of an African smoking "dakka" (1964:202-5).

Related to the neighboring Tswana we find the Sotho who occupy the present republic of Lesotho. One of the early missionaries who knew a great deal about these people described and diagrammed the pipe they used for smoking. He stated that "tobacco has long been in use among the natives, and must have come to them from the Portuguese of Mozambique but, in a song, consecrated to the praise of this favourite plant, they confess that the use of dagga (a kind of hemp, of which the Arabs make hagschisch), is much more ancient" (Casalis 1965:141). Much the

22

same position was taken by Nienaber who stated that the Khoikhoi smoked long before tobacco was introduced (1963:243). We are told that there was a time when the Sotho did not know tobacco, but they used to smoke hemp (Ellenberger and Macgregor 1912:9).

One of the ethnic groups on whom a great deal of information over a long period of time has been presented is the Zulu. They occupy most of Natal, and, as Nguni, are related to the Xhosa in the south and the Swazi in the north. John Bird, by referring to the subject twice, raises an interesting problem for us. He speaks first of "dakka" which according to him is "the dried leaf of the wild hemp," and indigenous to the country (1888:306). Later in the same volume we read of "sangu which is only European hemp, and raised for smoking." This is a problem, as suggested, because in most of the subsequent references and also in current usage, insangu is synonymous with dagga which is used to refer to *Cannabis sativa*. It would seem that we are back to the mistaken identity of dagga as "wild hemp" (see also Gardiner 1836:106, who suggested that the Zulu made a snuff of "dagga" leaves).

Writing even before Bird we find the reference of the Reverend Grout who spent half his lifetime among the Zulu. He speaks of smoking the pipe in which the bowl is filled "with the leaves and seed of the insangu" (1970:110). The Reverend Taylor (1891:122-23) wrote that "filthy and baneful" practice "[had] a narcotic and even intoxicating effect, similar to that of Indian hemp." He also is reminiscent of Latrobe's writing almost a century earlier in the Cape, when Latrobe suggested that smokers of hemp should be denied church membership (1969:159).

In a traditional Zulu community it was common for men to smoke insangu, even on a daily basis, and it seems that the effects were as varied as the individual personalities. Some smokers would exhibit extraordinary hilarity, others moroseness. It was especially at times of war that men would smoke the herb and, as saliva collects in the mouth, it would be passed through "a hollow stem of tambootie grass and so made to trace a labyrinth (tshuma sogexe) on a smooth floor" (Samuelson n.d.:81). The young warriors smoked cannabis before an attack and were then capable of accomplishing almost any feat. Bryant states that "the hemp (iNtsangu, *Cannabis sativa*) the Zulus smoked was home grown in every kraal" and that the best quality leaves were terminologically differentiated from the poorer kind (1949:222-23). In all these cases the traditional form of the pipe was used. The Zulu did not smoke tobacco as a rule but ground it into snuff. That is why they have only a single term for tobacco and snuff.

The Swazi used the cannabis pipe as well as the method by which a hole is made in the ground and the smoke sucked through a mouth-piece. The herb seems to have been associated here primarily with diviners who used a pipe. Following a puff of smoke each would fill his mouth with water to cool down the hot smoke (O'Neil 1921:307-9). It was also used as a stimulant by young warriors, as among the Zulu, and by the praise singer who must intone the praises of the king or some prominent person. It is contended by natives that the drug stimulates the brain. "If a man is faced with an extraordinary knotty problem he will smoke his shawulo (pipe) and concentrate on the problem and the solution will present itself to him without trouble" (Marwick 1940:80).

The water pipe, discussed in full later in this chapter, was found among all of these people. Slight variations obviously occurred as with the Venda, who did not, however, use cannabis very extensively (Stayt 1931:50-51). An identical description for the pipe as it was used by the Matabele is given by Decle (1898:24).

Since we suggested earlier that *Cannabis sativa* was introduced into Africa from the northeast, and not from the south as many suggest, it would be fruitful to follow briefly the pattern of its distribution and use. Dagga is a weed which in Zimbabwe can grow well only under cultivation. Thus the distribution of the plant must have been related to people. For normal growth it needs "a rich soil, fairly good rainfall and personal attention" (Editorial 1958:500). In Mashonaland it is known as Mbanji and is said to be a stimulus both sexually and in increasing work efficiency. It will be interesting to note how varied are the ascribed effects and contradictory the information among different authors.

With reference to the Tsonga of Mozambique we have some very good early descriptions by Junod (1927). This refers to the smoking of the drug, the saliva game which results, and the use of the herb in Tsonga ethnopharmacology. More recently Johnston (1975 and 1977) has illustrated the ritual use of cannabis as it is associated with beer drinking and young women's puberty initiation.

Having arrived at the great falls which he named after Queen Victoria, David Livingstone observed the smoking of cannabis among the Makololo, a Sotho offshoot. It is of interest that they called it Matokwane, as do the people of Lesotho. He describes its use as follows:

> We had ample opportunity for observing the effects of this matokwane smoking on our men. It makes them feel very strong in body, but it produces exactly the opposite effect upon the mind. Two of our finest young men became inveterate smokers, and partially idiotic. The performance of a group of matokwane smokers are somewhat grotesque; they are provided with a calabash of pure water, a split bamboo, five feet long, and the great pipe, which has a large calabash or kudu's horn chamber to contain the water, through which the smoke is drawn Narghille fashion, on its way to the mouth. Each smoker takes a few whiffs, the last being an extra long one, and hands the pipe to his neighbor. He seems to swallow the fumes; for, striving against the convulsive action of the muscles of chest and throat, he takes a mouthful of water from the calabash, waits a few seconds, and then pours water and smoke from his mouth down the groove of the bamboo. The smoke causes violent coughing in all, and in some a species of frenzy which passes away in a rapid stream of unmeaning words, or short sentences, as, 'the green grass grows,' 'the fat cattle thrive,' 'the fish swim.' (1865:286-87)

It was also used to give self-confidence to people, as in the case of the Zulu warriors mentioned earlier. Livingstone states that when the soldiers of the chief Sebitwane came in sight of their enemies, they "sat down and smoked it, in order that they might make an effective onslaught" (1857:540). Whatever hallucinogenic and stimulating properties may be present in cannabis, and whatever psychoactive material in Tetrahydrocannabinol (THC), it has long been recognized in the daily living by southern African people.

White immigrants. The white population group of South Africa derives primarily from early Dutch, French, and British settlers. The first Dutch settlement at what is now Cape Town was established in 1652 which at that time had no stage expansion and homesteading goals. In time, gardeners and cattle owners moved further from the fort, where the Dutch established a supply station for their ships sailing to and from the East, and finally were allowed to become free burghers. Since the route north and west from the settlement center took these early farmers into less fertile drier regions, their tendency was to claim farm land and graze their cattle along the east coast. In time they met and clashed with the southward migrating Nguni speakers and typical frontier skirmishes resulted.

Because Napoleon was expanding his influence in Europe, Britain decided to occupy the Cape and thus protect the eastern sea route. British occupation between 1795 and 1803 was uneventful, but when the British reoccupied the Cape on a permanent basis in 1806, they initiated major changes. These included a policy of social change which ultimately contributed to the Great Trek—a major population movement by White frontiersmen into the interior. It is their descendants who emerged as the Afrikaners.

The province of Natal in which Durban is located was originally inhabited by Africans of the Nguni linguistic group as discussed above. In 1823 the British occupied the natural harbour and called it Port Natal. As the settlement grew and British administration of the Cape became more permanent, one of the governors of the Cape Colony, Sir Benjamin D'Urban, was later honored by the renaming of this port settlement after him. Across the Drakensburg range in the interior at this time came the first of the Boer frontiersmen as they sought to settle the grassy plains of what they saw as an unclaimed region.

As a consequence of policy clashes between the local Voortrekker Volksraad and the British government in the Cape in 1842, the British sent a regiment to occupy Port Natal. In 1844 the port and an area to be known as Natal were annexed to the Cape Colony and British administration was extended over the region from the Indian Ocean to the Drakensburg range. Natal at this time had a population of about 100,000 Blacks and 3,000 Whites. The latter were widely dispersed between the Tugela River in the north and the Umzinkulu River in the south, and inland to the Afrikaner settlements of Weenen, Utrecht, Vryheid and surrounding farms.

Soon British settlers were residing in Durban and gentlemen farmers were growing sugar in ever increasing acres of fertile coastal land. After a few years sugar mills were constructed and in 1860, barely five years after the first local sale of Natal sugar, the young industry exported its first full cargo of 250 bags of sugar to England. Port Natal (Durban) developed into a major port and city.

Sugarcane cultivation and sugar refining also opened up industry and major employment possibilities for the indigenous African population. Africans were unwilling to leave their own lands in order to work alien lands and crops for wages and failed to seize these job opportunities. As a result East Indian laborers under a system of indenture were brought to Natal in order to cultivate the sugarcane fields and work in the refineries. The first Indian coolies arrived aboard the *Truro* on 16 November 1860, some to return at the end of their indentures and some to stay. Those who stayed permanently changed not only the face of Durban and Natal but also of the whole of South Africa.

The Coloured population. Marais differentiates three periods of history for the Coloureds up to 1937. The first extends from 1652, when the Whites began to settle in the region, to 1838 when legal discrimination against Khoikhoi and Coloureds ended for a short while. The second period, the laissez-faire phase mentioned above, reaches from 1838 to 1920 during which the Coloureds were legally equal and allowed to work and live freely among the Whites. It was during this phase that the St. Helenans and the Mauritians came to Durban hoping to better their economic and social status. Not until the end of the second Boer War, in 1902, did the steady growth of the sentiments that are basic to apartheid clearly turn against the Coloureds. Up to that time, the Coloureds had avoided the discrimination leveled at the Indians and the Blacks. The Coloureds had retained the franchise that had been taken from the Indians in 1893, and their children were able to attend White government schools. And yet, harbingers of apartheid were present. Social discrimination existed, and often controversy emerged over the St. Helenan children being in the same classes as Whites. It becomes apparent that the Coloureds were only initially unaffected by White prejudice because of their cultural similarity and small numbers. It was only a matter of time for change to occur. By 1920, the beginning of the third phase was well underway. The State began the process whereby Coloureds would be excluded from competition against Whites for the better occupations. By 1948, the political domination of the Afrikaners was assured through the Nationalist party that acted to legislate apartheid into every facet of the life of the Coloured.

Culturally the Durban Coloureds are very different from the Cape Province Coloureds. Eighty-two percent of Durban Coloureds speak English at home while 90 percent of Cape Province Coloureds speak Afrikaans at home. Forty-three percent of the Durbanites are Roman Catholic compared to 70 percent of those in the Cape Province. Nine percent of the Durbanites are members of the Dutch Reformed Church while 29 percent of those in the Cape Province belong to this church. The Coloured population of Durban is a small minority accounting for approximately 4 percent of the city's population. The first representatives of this group were the produce of crosses between Europeans, Malay slaves and Blacks. Unlike the Cape Province Coloureds, they lack a Khoikhoi strain and have a relatively small Malay admixture. In other Coloured groups, Malay-European unions were most frequent as White-Bengal slave marriages began in 1656, shortly after the first colonialization of South Africa (Dickie-Clark 1966:50). However, products of these relations represent a small dispersed group in Durban. The first large concentration of Coloureds was composed of the Mauritians who migrated into Durban in 1850 to work in the sugar industry. These individuals were skilled artisans who were Western by culture, and thus very similar to the Whites of Durban. A smaller group of St. Helenans also migrated into the city at this time. They had been domestic servants on St. Helena and were thus also Westernized.

The large number of English-speaking Coloureds in Durban is the result of the long history of British domination of Natal. Durban Coloureds are different from Cape Province Coloureds in other ways as well. They are less rigorously segregated and better off economically. Dickie-Clark estimates that on an annual basis they may earn up to twice as much as Cape Coloureds. In addition, the absence of any subculture is notable. Among the Cape

Province populations, a distinctive dialect of Afrikaans has emerged, and the Coons Carnival tradition has become established. These elements, or ones that are comparable, may yet appear in the Durban population, as the trend in all South African urban centers is toward parallel or separate development. Currently, however, there is little cultural difference between Whites and Coloureds in Durban.

The Durban Coloureds are similar to the Whites culturally, even though they are now socially, politically, and economically only slightly above the Indians and Blacks in terms of status. In spite of their subordinate role, they continue to identify with the Whites and with White culture. A marked bias in favor of Whites and a certain prejudice against Blacks and Indians have been observed. They think of themselves as possessing White genes and aim to maintain "a decent, White" standard of living. The ambiguity of their situation, the marginality of their group as Dickie-Clark describes it, has led to a certain amount of isolation. The Coloureds are included in a hierarchy in which the strata are incompletely separated from each other (Dickie-Clark 1966:153). They have attempted to emphasize those characteristics that are similar to the White's and deemphasize those that are similar to the Indian's and Black's in order to clarify their inconsistent status to their own advantage. However, the Whites continue to avoid interacting with them, and the Coloureds avoid interacting with the Blacks and Indians as their dominant position over these groups is no longer clear.

The Coloureds have some of the same rights and privileges as the Whites. They have better educational facilities at their disposal than are available for the Indians and Blacks. They had basically the same civil rights as the Whites in terms of movement and freedom of thought, religion, public expression, and association until a number of acts and amendments of acts in the 1960s and 1970s affected everyone. In the past they were politically better represented than the Blacks and Indians. It was not until 1956 that they were removed from the common voting roll and even then 500 Durban Coloured men were allowed to continue to vote until 1960 when the Referendum Act No. 52, forbade non-Whites from voting in the Republican referendum. Currently, they only have the right to be represented in the Coloured

Representation Council which was established by Proclamation 77 in 1969.

In spite of certain advantages Coloureds continue to have over the Indians and Blacks, they have been seriously affected by such apartheid legislation as the Group Areas Act No. 41. This law, passed in 1950, reserves occupancy and ownership of particular areas to people of certain ethnic identity. Through this law, the poor and low-cost housing has been parceled out to the Coloureds. In 1961, approximately 20 percent of Durban's Coloureds were living in one of the three segregated housing projects reserved for them. In addition, far less money is spent annually on the education of Coloured children than is spent on a White child's education. One might expect from the unique history of frustrated opportunities that the Coloured population of Durban experienced that a certain amount of hostility exists. How this hostility is channelled is beyond the scope of this study.

Above we have established the Coloured population within South African culture, but we have also qualified this statement by introducing Dickie-Clark's theory that the Coloureds are a marginal society within this greater unit. If we accept this premise and agree that the Coloureds are a separate society, then it follows that the component individuals in this society have evolved an organized behavior as well as a group consciousness, a feeling of unity (Linton 1936:92-93). This adaptation of individuals through behavior and attitudes held in common enables the group to function as a unit. Yet, even in the most isolated situations, new conditions arise that entail creative responses on the part of the component individual (Linton 1936:95). A new adaptation, through language and close contact, can spread quickly through the society or be transmitted first to one group and then more gradually to the rest of society.

The speed with which change in attitudes occurs is often closely related to the focus of the socialization process. To better understand the relative importance of such institutions as kinship, nonkinship social groups such as peers, economy, politics, and religion to the Coloured population in Durban, we would like to establish our sample within a transitional phase between what Riesman would describe as an inner-directed type of individual and an other-directed type of person (Riesman 1950:15,19-22).

30

Riesman correlates demographic factors, such as high population growth and urbanization, with certain social characteristics (Riesman 1952:8-9). Character here is defined as those components of personality that play an important part in the maintenance of social forms. For the most part, these are learned so that, as Fromm stated, man will desire to act in the way that he must act according to society (Fromm 1944:381).

Inner-directed character types are found in societies that are undergoing an increase in population, an increase in personal mobility, a rapid accumulation of capital, and an expansion of goods. Because of the above factors, it becomes necessary for individuals to be able to make certain choices about their future based upon internalized controls that were instilled in them as children by parents and other important adult authorities (Riesman 1952:6). Thus, even though tradition is still important (to the inner-directed society) in that it limits the individual's choices and his means of attaining these ends, a new flexibility appears, helping people cope with the novelties the quickly changing world affords.

Other-directed behavior character types are found in societies of incipient population decline or those cultures where the birth and death rates are equal, anticipating the time when the birth rate will drop below the death rate. In these societies tertiary occupations, or services and nonproductive activities, become increasingly important. In addition to this shift in emphasis, a sensitivity to the quality of interpersonal relations appears. This sensitivity to peers and to others provides the main source of direction for people within this society. They obey a fluctuating list of short-term goals that are dictated by the contemporaries of the individual.

We would like to establish the Coloureds of our sample within the transition phase between the above two types of society. Overlapping is not uncommon in any nation as there can be a number of different sectors in any one area, each exemplifying one of the three character types Riesman describes (1950:31). Thus, in South Africa, it would not be unusual for tradition-directed individuals to exist in the rural areas, inner-directed individuals to be common in the urban Black or Coloured populations, and other-directed peoples to exist in the urban Coloured or White groups. In addition, a number of groups, of any ethnic identity, might exist in the transition state between the two character types.

31

The Coloureds in our sample are one example of this. In many ways they appear to be part of an inner-directed society. Their families are large, and their population is very young compared to other South African ethnic groups. In many ways for them, their parents are models of absolute authority. As we will see later concerning the attitudes of family and household members, the parents are convinced that their ideals and values are the right ones. Since that is the case their offspring's cannabis habit represents some failure on the parents' part. Both are tested and compared to ideals in their perfection, absolute standards that the parents adhere to consistently. Families involved do not automatically embrace new trends and values as they present themselves. Rather they have certain basic standards that they refuse to relinquish.

Economically, the Coloureds in our sample also seem to fit into the ideal inner-directed society described by Riesman. They are not part of the upper-income category though they are better off financially than the Blacks. They are employed in jobs that require workmen skills and qualities, and not finer human relations and cooperation (Riesman 1950:115). They still are part of the working class.

However, the Coloureds are taking on many of the characteristics of an other-directed society. Though their families are still large and their population young, they do not live in extended families. Rather, the offspring live with the parents alone in an atmosphere that has the potential for intense personal relations that will sensitize the child to human interactional problems. This sensitivity opens the child to new influences. His peer group becomes increasingly important so that the parents no longer represent absolute authority to them. Rather, the maturity of his friends takes on new proportions, and the individual gradually becomes, what Riesman calls, other-directed. We will see that this indeed is what has happened to the Coloureds in our sample. "Becoming one of the gang" and being included in the cannabis network are very valuable to the individual. What this group does and how it views cannabis and other experiences becomes increasingly important to those questioned. Values and standards are drawn from new and more varied sources than before.

Changes are also occurring in the economic sector. For example, the Coloureds live in urban centers, traditionally the source of other-directed character (Riesman 1950:114). Their coworkers, as friends and companions, are a new variable in their job patterns. The large number that considered their coworkers as friends (see discussion below) attests to the fact that the Coloured person does not work in isolation. He is no longer as job-oriented as he was in the past. Instead he currently interacts with his peers and with his supervisor in a social manner.

The Indians of Natal. When the Republic of Natalia was annexed by Great Britain in 1843, it became a district of the Cape Colony and thus subject to direct British administration. Most of the Boer frontiersmen left during the following five years and their places were taken by some 5,000 European, mostly British, settlers. The arrival of the Europeans and their subsequent economic initiatives, particularly in the expansion of the sugar industry, created a need for laborers who at that time could not be obtained locally.

A public meeting was held in Durban in October 1851 to discuss this most critical need. Various solutions were debated including the importation of laborers from the East, but no definite steps were taken. Four years later in 1855, Sir George Grey, who had recently been appointed Governor of the Cape Colony (and thus High Commissioner for Natal), visited Natal. On a visit to a sugar estate the question of labor was brought up and Grey expressed his preference for Indian rather than Chinese laborers. Both nationalities had been used extensively in other parts of the world under British control. Indians were used as indentured laborers in many sugar producing colonies such as British Guiana, Mauritius, Fiji and the West Indies, especially Trinidad. With the dissolution of the English East India Company in 1858, the peoples of India came under the direct control of the British Government.

Upon Grey's recommendation, the British Government, both in England and India, eventually agreed to such a transfer of laborers. Natal Law No. 14 which dealt with the introduction of laborers from India, and Natal Law No. 15 making it possible for persons to import (at their own expense) immigrants from India, were soon promulgated by the Natal government. In 1860, the Indian Act XXXIII was passed permitting the emigration of Indian laborers to Natal, and on October 12 of that year the first ship, the *Truro*, sailed from Madras. Most of the early recruits were from the Madras Presidency and were pariahs. In addition, Indian

33

laborers also came from Upper Pradesh, Madhya Pradesh, Orissa, Western Bengal and the Northern and North Eastern districts. Later migrants, the so-called passenger Indians, came from Kathiawar, Porbandar, and Surat, as well as from Bombay and the northern provinces. Their numbers, however, were relatively small. A few were Muslims while a small number belonged to the Sudra Caste. During the next six years more than six thousand laborers left Madras and Calcutta. Between 1866 and 1874 emigration was temporarily held up while the living conditions of Indian migrants in Natal were being inspected (Kondapi 1951:21).

Most of the Indian recruits belonged to the agricultural class, and the epithet coolie in time became a derogatory term used by both English- and Afrikaans-speaking South Africans of different colors. While these Indian workers were originally imported to work on sugar plantations, they abandoned them at the end of their indentures and were soon employed in the dockyards and railways in Durban, in the coal mines further inland, on smallholder gardens, and in domestic employment and municipal service. Few ever saw the country of their birth again.

The diversification of lifestyles which began to emerge is described clearly by Chattopadhyaya. Quoting first from the annual report for 1874-1875 by the Protector of Immigrants in Natal, Colonel B. P. Lloyd, Chattopadhyaya stated as follows:

While between 7 and 8 thousand (Indians in Natal) are employed on the estates along the coast, the remainder are scattered over the colony in various capacities as domestic servants, traders, storekeepers, market-gardeners, boatmen, fishermen, etc. The Indians still enjoy a monopoly of the fish trade, and a very large proportion of the vegetables and not a little of the fruits, consumed by the Europeans in the town of Maritzburg and Durban, are grown by them. They are rapidly acquiring land and many are now competing with their masters in agricultural pursuits. I am of the opinion that the coolies hold over 1,000 acres of land in the Manda division alone. They pay on an average of £1 per acre per annum and are most industrious, working morning, noon and night.

34

He continued, quoting from the report of the Natal Economic Commission of 1814:

> The indentured Indian of the early days, when his term of service expired, often took up land and grew vegetables, mealies and tobacco. To a certain extent, he reindentured and took service with Europeans, but of late years he has increasingly entered the semi-skilled trades. Today he is engaged in the building trades, printing, boot-repairing, tailoring, painting, mattress-making and other miscellaneous callings of the semi-skilled trades. Many so engaged are Natal-born Indians, and numbers who speak English are employed as cooks, waiters, drivers, vanmen, and in lawyers' offices, as junior clerks and touts. (Chattopadhyaya 1970:66)

After the temporary halt of emigration between 1866 and 1874, indenturing was resumed and continued until 1911. Kuper (1960) found that from 1883 to 1890, 11,501 persons sailed for Natal from Madras and 4,925 from Calcutta. By 1911, though, the largest proportion of the original laborers had left the sugar plantations and had become "free" Indians. Some did return to India under a government sponsored repatriation scheme, which included a cash bonus, but the majority became permanent residents of South Africa.

In addition to the indentured laborers a large number of free passenger Indians migrated to Natal. These were persons who came under the ordinary immigration law, paying their own way and enjoying citizenship rights until these were changed (Pachai 1971). The immigrants had a commercial motive and nearly all went into business in Natal and Transvaal. Such persons were mostly Muslims speaking Guzerati or Urdu along with some Hindus. Parsees from Bombay, Zoroastrians by religion, formed a smaller group.

It is with the first group, the indentured laborers who in time became free Indians, that we are here primarily concerned. At the time that Indians were migrating to Natal, the Indian government was deeply involved in an investigation of cannabis use throughout the country. The report of these investigations refers to use and users by geographical district. Thus, once the districts of origin could be fixed it became possible for us to reconstruct drug use patterns in India according to the regions from which migrants derived and to compare drug use patterns in India and Natal. The Report of the Indian Hemp Drugs Commission (1894) comprises seven volumes and 3,281 pages. It ranks with the most complete and systematic surveys of cannabis to date.

The Indian laborers who migrated to Natal, therefore, must have been familiar with the handling of the cannabis plant both in the spontaneous and the cultivated form. Upon their arrival in Natal they were bound to encounter cannabis growing with great abundance and their familiarity with it may have influenced their attitude toward an herb identified, at that time, with the indigenous Black population. Having come from areas where they could observe such preparations going on, the Indian migrants to Natal would have had little difficulty in adjusting themselves to conditions in coastal Natal. The living conditions to which these Indian laborers migrated allowed for much the same lifestyle. Most of them went to rural settings where they had their own gardens and adjacent uncultivated areas. They also had private homes or compound facilities where the herb, if grown could be matured and prepared.

When the *Truro* and all other subsequent laborer-carrying ships discharged their cargo at Durban, they left behind Indian workers who retained an Indian homogeneity. Their ethnic identity, appearance, religions and languages set them off from the English-speaking gentlemen farmers—most of whom came from Britain—and the dark-skinned Zulu-speakers, dressed in traditional costume. Being uneducated and relatively unsophisticated, as well as being laborers, these Indians should have had greater contact with the Zulu—who were beginning to enter the labor market and who resided throughout the district—than with the Whites. Though documentation is lacking, we would also expect that they established supply networks of cannabis and later of opium within a short time after landing in Natal.

Ten years after the first Indian indentured laborers arrived in Natal, Law No. 2, 1870, known as the "Coolie Law Consolidation," was passed. One section of paragraph 70 states that the purpose connected with the law is "prohibiting the smoking, use, or possession by and the sale, barter, or gift to, any Coolies whatsoever, of any portion of the hemp plant (Cannabis sativa); and authorizing the destruction thereof, if found in such use or possession; and imposing penalties upon Coolies using, cultivating, or possessing such plant for the purpose of smoking the same." This law did not, however, greatly affect a cultural pattern as well established as cannabis use. We should also note that this law speaks of sales to Indians but not of the cultivation by Indians of their own cannabis plants.

In July 1884, the Natal Legislative Council appointed a commission under the chairmanship of Walter Wragg, a Supreme Court judge, to report on the Indian Immigration Laws and Regulations of the Colony, and on the general condition of the Indian population in Natal. Known locally as the Wragg Commission it reported back to the Council in 1887. The second chapter of the report discusses cannabis in relation to Indians.

The third section of Chapter II says that "hemp is cultivated by Indian Immigrants and by Kaffirs; in many parts of the Colony it grows wild." Within little over a decade the Indian laborers had resumed cannabis cultivation as had been their wont in India. Most of them smoked it but "other Indians consume a mixture compounded of tobacco, opium, hemp, and brown sugar. The fumes from this compound [were] not even passed through water to abstract the volatile oils and cannabis resin" (1887:6—sic). Though we now know that cannabinols are not water soluble so that the water pipe merely cools the smoke, it is significant that Indians were smoking the same mixture as was usual in India.

The report then turns to section 70 of Law 2 of 1870, where it pointed out that the word "sativa" was used to indicate the cultivated, as contrasted with the wild, variety of hemp. The Commission members concluded, however, that immoderate use of cannabis was dangerous, detrimental to the health of the smoker, led to crime, and rendered the Indian immigrant unfit and unable to perform. They recommended, therefore, that section 70 of Law 2 of 1870 be changed to read as follows:

1. Prohibiting the cultivation, by Indian Immigrants, of any variety of cannabis, the hemp plant
2. Prohibiting the smoking or the possession, by Indian Immigrants, of any portion of the hemp plant, whether

wild or cultivated, save by medical advice, the proof whereof shall be on the smoker or possessor

3. Prohibiting the sale to Indian immigrants, of any portion of the hemp plant, whether wild or cultivated, by any person other than a duly license vendor, who shall require, before such sale, the production of a satisfactory certificate

4. Imposing a stamp duty upon all licenses issued under the rules

5. Authorizing the destruction of any variety of the hemp plant, cultivated by or found, without authority, in possession of Indian immigrants, by order of the Resident Magistrate of the district

6. Imposing penalties, not exceeding two pounds, for any breach of such rules (1887:7)

It is of interest that neither the law of 1870 nor the report of 1887 mentioned any mode of cannabis use other than smoking. The liquids, sweetmeats, resin extracts and other forms of the drug were ignored, indicating that the leaves were smoked in the same way the Zulu did.

We should not consider, however, that the Indians and Zulu were acting independently of each other or of Whites. Even at that time interethnic networks existed, such as they do today. This point is acknowledged in the Commission's report which recognized the role of White traders, Zulu growers, and Indian users.

We have reason to think that much hemp is sold to Indians by Kaffirs and storekeepers; we are aware that in some parts of the Colony, white traders purchase green hemp leaves from Kaffir growers and retail them, in a dried state, to any customer who applies for them. As we are strongly convinced that the smoking of hemp is as baneful to the Kaffir as to the Indian, we consider that it is our duty to suggest that chemists, holding special licenses subject to stamp duty, should be the only persons allowed by law to sell any portion of the hemp plant, whether wild or cultivated, to any person whomsoever, whether of White, Kaffir, or Indian descent." (1887:8)

In time, Indian laborers became settlers, farmers, business-men, and professionals. In 1960 about 8.6 percent of the economically active Indian population were still employed in agriculture. By 1970 this figure had declined to 3.7 percent. Many of this segment of the population are growers of cannabis, others are suppliers. A significant number of Indians today smoke cannabis.

In 1985 the Indian population of South Africa was about 820,000—the largest group of Indians outside the Indian sub-continent and Sri Lanka. Of these, 660,000 or 80 percent lived in the province of Natal, the majority within a radius of ninety-five miles of Durban. Since most of the indentured laborers of the nineteenth century were Hindus (70 percent), their descendants are divided into four linguistic groups speaking Tamil, Telugu, Hindustani, or Gujerati. Muslims (comprising 20 percent of the Indian population) speak mostly Urdu or Gujerati. The Gujerati are about three-fourths Muslim and one-fourth Hindu.

The South African Indian community has retained group coherence. The family is a strong unit and religion unites parents and children to a greater degree than is evident in other ethnic groups. A ban on the use of alcohol in both the Hindu and Islamic religion (Balkisson 1973:6-7) has not prevented it being accepted nowadays by many in the community. Yet despite such seculariza-tion, Indian women rarely smoke or use alcohol. According to one author (Meer 1969:71) and from personal observation, two cate-gories have to be included. Elderly women among the peasant and working class families have appropriated and are granted the masculine right to smoke and drink. The same permissiveness pertains to Westernized women who have attained a high profes-sional status. It is to be expected, for example, that among female university students who are both secularized and aspire to a professional career, there would also be persons who use alcohol and possibly cannabis.

These, then, are the four ethnic groups, legally distinguished which make up this study. Three of the groups are immigrants into South Africa: first the Blacks, then the Whites, and finally, the Indians. In many ways the Coloureds are the most South African of all four categories of this sample. They had their origin in South Africa, they derive from no other region, and they are genetically related to all the other groups. While the Indians have remained relatively "pure" they have contributed genetically, culturally and religiously to the Coloured population in Natal.

The study

During the 1970s there was a growing concern about drug use in the United States as well as an interest in what could be learned from cross-cultural studies. Part of this concern and interest focused on cannabis. The concern over cannabis and its possible effects, both immediate and long term, prompted the National Institute on Mental Health in Washington to establish the National Institute on Drug Abuse (NIDA). Rather than fund only studies in the U.S. where drug use was artificial and the drug frequently imported, the NIDA funded a number of international studies which looked at chronic cannabis use in its natural setting. What further differentiated these latter studies is that they looked at drug use in the normal social context rather than focus on persons who had been institutionalized or incarcerated.

It was in this context that our project on cannabis use in Africa, with actual field study in South Africa, was approached. The research focused on all four of the major ethnic groups in South Africa; though concentrating on the use of cannabis, we expanded the study to look at other drugs.

As part of this overall study of drug use, particularly cannabis smoking in the Natal region of South Africa, it was decided to include high school pupils, namely twelfth graders, in this research. A questionnaire was compiled to study aspects of drug use and attitudes regarding drugs among this sample of South African adolescents. It was composed of five major sections:

1. Social background
2. History of cannabis use
3. Social aspects influencing use, e.g., friends, parents, and values
4. Attitudes regarding cannabis, its effects, its legal status, etc.
5. Use of and attitudes regarding other drugs

With permission of various Departments of Education, the questionnaire was administered to senior students at twelve high schools in and around Durban during April 1974. Eleven years later, during April 1985, it was possible to visit eleven of the same schools and administer essentially the same questionnaire to the senior students. The one exception was a Black school which had arranged a special teachers' workday on short notice. This restudy permits us to record changes in attitudes about and frequency of drug use over a decade—all the more significant because it involves the four major ethnic classifications recognized by South African law and pertains to a time of rapid internal change in that country.

Table 1 represents the students included in the two studies at the same schools. It is important to understand that these schools are all ethnically segregated and located in segregated residential neighborhoods. In the case of the White schools, the coeducational English medium school is on the city outskirts, while the boys' and girls' schools are both prestigious schools in a wealthy and exclusive neighborhood in Durban.

Table 1

ETHNIC COMPOSITION OF TWO STUDENT
RESEARCH SAMPLES

High Schools	1974	1985
Black (two schools)*	228	126
Coloured (three schools)	89	180
Indian (three schools)	337	341
White: Afrikaans medium	88	82
English medium co-ed	119	132
English medium boys	146	90
English medium girls	145	108
TOTAL	1,152	1,059

*In 1985, only one Black school was visited.

41

On both occasions, the questionnaire was presented to the students in complete privacy and without either teachers or school administrators in attendance. The students had the researcher's assurance of complete anonymity. The results are as close to a true and honest reflection of drug attitudes and patterns of use among school students as was possible to attain under the circumstances.

Summary

The discussion which follows concerns drug use among South African high school students. It focuses on their family backgrounds, their peer groups, their attitudes, and their religious and social involvement. Since we are dealing with a questionnaire as survey instrument and a large sample, the presentation will necessarily involve a degree of quantification in the form of comparative tables.

3

DEMOGRAPHIC BACKGROUND OF THE SOUTH AFRICAN ADOLESCENT STUDY SAMPLE

Introduction

Matriculation, Senior Certificate, Form Five, or Standard Ten, as the final year in high school is variously termed marks the point at which schooling in South Africa is terminated. After graduation a relatively small percentage of Blacks, Coloureds, and Indians go to the university, whereas a much larger percentage of Whites do so. For many it is the end of financial security if their parents have been able to support them, and so the last year in high school is important. The student has become one of the older members in school, with better access to sports teams, debating societies, and the like. These are the students who wear their school colors with pride, reflecting in many cases athletic achievements. Rather than deal with the different ethnic groups, we will discuss the material in terms of various topics.

In the demographic data the relatively favorable condition of the Whites will immediately be evident. This reflects not only their economic conditions at the times of these surveys but shows White students as products of better socioeconomic and educational traditions. Because of color barriers, social class and caste are self-perpetuating.

Age

Age of first schooling, proximity of schools, financial ability to remain in school, and the quality of schools and teachers all are reflected in the age of students at certain levels of schooling. In favorable conditions children start day school at age six and would be in the final year of their twelve years of public schooling at age seventeen, higher if a student had to repeat a year or had started school at a later age.

In the 1974 survey it was found that the relative age of students in their final year of high school was significantly lower for White, Coloured and Indian as compared to Black. This is confirmed in the 1985 figures (Table 2 and Chart): 94.2 percent of the White, 80.6 percent of the Coloured, and 86.8 percent of the Indian students are below eighteen years of age, compared to only 24 percent of the Black students. It is obvious that socioeconomic factors are at work as are factors regarding housing, distance from schools, and possibly quality of education as students might be required to repeat a year.

Table 2

AGE OF HIGH SCHOOL SENIORS
BY ETHNIC GROUP

Age	Black		Coloured		Indian		White	
	No.	%	No.	%	No.	%	No.	%
16	4	3.2	5	2.8	1	0.3	15	3.6
17	8	6.4	66	36.7	146	42.8	209	50.7
18	18	14.4	74	41.1	149	43.7	164	39.8
19	35	28.0	24	13.3	34	10.0	21	5.1
20	30	24.0	10	5.6	10	2.9	3	0.7
21	18	14.4	1	0.6	1	0.3	-	-
22	7	5.6	-	-	-	-	-	-
23+	5	4.0	-	-	-	-	-	-
Total	125	100.0	180	100.1	341	100.0	412	99.9

Sex

Normally in most countries the ratio of male students to female students will be purely incidental or may reflect the birth patterns of a particular group or a particular era. However, in South African, we are dealing with an interesting cultural value ascribed to education by Indians. Among Black, Coloured, and White South Africans, there was no significant pattern in the ratio

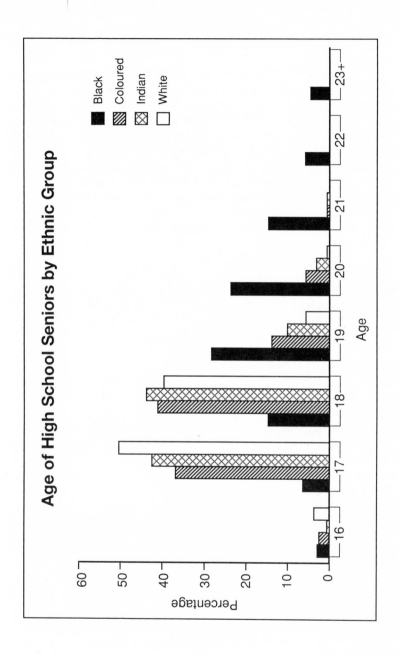

Age of High School Seniors by Ethnic Group

of male to female students. Where males might have been in the majority in 1974, the reverse might be true in 1985.

Traditionally, Indian families have placed great value on the education and qualifications of their sons. Families were strongly patriarchal; the father (and father's brothers) made decisions affecting minors, that is women and children. The father was also responsible for the morals of his children; to assure a successful marriage he had to protect daughters from even a hint of scandal. The result was that girls were allowed to go to school, even coeducational schools, but upon reaching menarche, they were summarily withdrawn and kept home to await an acceptable match. In some cases they were permitted to go to girls' schools (du Toit 1990). In a changing society the extended family has decreased in its importance and the status of women, both as companions and economic partners, has increased. By 1985, and this was a recent phenomenon, Indian South African girls and young women were conspicuous in high schools, teachers' colleges and universities. This change is also evident in these studies. In 1974 the school population was only 44.0 percent girls, but the figure rose to 49.5 percent of students ten years later.

Language

Because the students in the sample belonged to different ethnic groups, they also represented different language groups. The percentage of students claiming a particular home language does reflect on the South African demographic and cultural matrix. The Durban region in the province of Natal is historically an area associated with the Zulu tribal group and thus with speakers of the Zulu language. It is not strange to find a relatively stable Black population of whom 93.9 percent spoke Zulu as its home language in 1974 and 92.8 percent in 1985. As urbanization and particularly urban residence increased, it was more common to find interethnic marriages, Zulu-speakers with other language group members or educated couples who prefer to speak English at home.

Into this province of Natal came British settlers who in time developed vast sugar plantations as well as other industries. When the Union of South Africa was formed in 1910, Natal was the most British and "English" of the four provinces. Even today this is true—particularly in the port city of Durban—and this predominance is reflected in the home language of students. In 1974 78.9 percent indicated English and 18.1 percent indicated Afrikaans as their home language. In 1985 these figures changed only slightly, as 78.2 percent versus 20.4 percent indicated the two official languages as their home languages. The slight gain in Afrikaans is at the expense of "other" (indicating immigrants) and represents a concerted effort by Afrikaner cultural and economic organizations and the Nationalist party to strengthen the status of Afrikaners in Durban.

Historically, the Indians were the third group to enter Natal when they were brought in after 1860 as indentured laborers. Caste groups broke down, but marriages continued to be within linguistic and especially religious groups. The family remained the strongest and most conservative institution within which linguistic, and religious traditions were perpetuated. Secularism, particularly within the last two or three decades has resulted in a breakdown of family authority in reference groups outside the family, in education of daughters, and thus in linguistic and religious group heterogeneity. We find that among the Indians, the percentage of students who claimed English as their home language increased from 46.1 percent to 86.2 percent in the ten year interval. This growth was at the expense of traditional Indian languages which respectively decreased, in the case of Tamil, from 22.6 percent to 8.5 percent; Hindi, from 12.8 percent to 1.5 percent; Urdu, from 8.3 percent to 1.8 percent; Gujerati, from 3.6 percent to .3 percent; and "other" (which includes Telegu and Arabic), from 3.6 percent to 1.8 percent. All these figures point at the acceptance of English as the standard language, with most of the younger generation becoming passive-bilingual, that is they understand their mother tongue and may be able to read it but cannot speak it.

The last group, the Coloureds, are nationally recognized as being identified with the Afrikaans language as well as Afrikaner religious and cultural expressions. In the case of the Coloureds in Natal, there was a much stronger English identification, and perhaps as a result of political developments a degree of anti-Afrikaans sentiment. This was also reflected in the home language of students. Those who claimed English increased from 89.9 percent in 1974 to 97.2 percent in 1985. This change was at the expense of those claiming Afrikaans as their home language, which decreased from 10.1 percent to 2.8 percent over the ten year period.

Future plans

I would venture that the socioeconomic status and freedom of individuals are no better measured than by their future plans and aspirations, which might reflect dreams or ideals or represent the realities of restrictions and imposed limitations. They may, of course, also reflect acceptance of economic realities.

When this survey was first conducted in 1974, Blacks in the Durban area had only two possibilities for tertiary education—attending a segregated Black university, almost certainly the University of Zululand, or studying by correspondence through the University of South Africa. Advanced postgraduate students could enroll in medical school at the University of Natal. Between 1974 and 1985 two major changes had occurred: the establishment of a network of technicons, schools based on the model of the American community colleges, and the integration of tertiary education by the "opening" of universities. Opening technically permitted a Black student to attend the University of Natal (previously all White) or the University of Durban-Westville (previously restricted to Indians). Coloureds could travel to the Cape to attend the University of the Western Cape, go to Bechet Teachers' Training College in Durban, or enroll in the University of Natal Medical School. The same avenue was open to medical students who were Indian, but the majority of these attended the University of Durban-Westville. For the White high school senior, there was the choice of ten universities and an equal number of teachers' training colleges. For all ethnic groups, there was the possibility of technical college or the option of going to work. In spite of high aspirations and ideals, economics frequently forced a choice upon the student.

Contrary to the relatively small number of Black students who attended a university, a very large number aspired to tertiary education—an alternative to going to work. In the color-caste based South African society, Black workers have the most difficult time, socially and economically. In the light of these facts, it was of interest to find that Black high schools had the highest percentage of students who hoped to attend a university or teacher

48

training college and the lowest percentage who wanted to go to work.

Table 3 suggests that the relative position of the different ethnic groups did not change between 1974 and 1985. Black students remained those who most aspired to study and least planned to go to work. Although the figures for universities were down, a larger number planned to train as teachers or to attend a technicon which will give them a skill.

Religion

Religious group membership or identification does not imply participation or religiosity. Religiosity has been found to be associated with drug exposure and experimentation, but the latter has not been found to be correlated with a particular denomination. Religion in the South African context has taken on certain political overtones while also reflecting historical traditions.

Among Black South Africans, traditional animists were the subject of intense missionary endeavors by a vast array of European churches and evangelical groups. Such activity produced Black Christians of every conceivable denomination, but it also led to expressions of independence or opposition. Thus there emerged a range of independent churches which have been classified as being either Zionistic or Ethiopean in their conception and teaching or Messianic in their futuristic orientation. These separatist churches are today one of the most numerous categories on the religious horizon in South Africa.

Hindus and Muslims are almost exclusively restricted to Indian South Africans. It is interesting that the 1980 population census reports religious group membership in Natal as being 71.9 percent Hindu and 14.0 percent Muslim (the latter are much more numerous in Transvaal). Table 4 confirms this relative strength among the student population. When we turn to religious participation or attendance at worship services, we once again face a problem, because Hindus normally do not "go to church." Home worship, lighting of the lamps, and similar activities are practiced instead. When we were told that among Indian students the most frequent form of religious expression was attendance on religious holy days only, the result must be seen in context.

49

Table 3
PLANS AND ASPIRATIONS OF HIGH SCHOOL SENIORS

Choice	Black				Coloured				Indian				White			
	1974		1985		1974		1985		1974		1985		1974		1985	
	No.	%	No.	%	No.	%	No.	%	No.	%	No.	%	No.	%	No.	%
Go to university	132	58.4	48	38.7	33	38.0	22	12.3	103	30.7	100	29.5	219	44.0	133	32.4
Go to teacher's college	27	11.9	42	33.9	6	6.7	43	24.0	40	11.9	27	8.0	49	9.8	25	6.1
Go to technicon	-	-	25	20.2	-	-	55	30.7	-	-	79	23.3	-	-	75	18.2
Go to work	21	9.3	3	2.4	15	17.3	13	7.3	58	17.3	58	17.1	59	11.8	46	11.2
Other and undecided	46	20.4	6	4.8	33	38.0	46	25.7	135	40.1	75	22.2	171	34.4	132	32.1
Total	226	100.0	124	100.0	87	100.0	179	100.0	336	100.0	339	100.0	498	100.0	411	100.0
No response	2		2		2		1		1		2		1		1	

50

Table 4

RELIGIOUS GROUP OR DENOMINATIONAL AFFILIATION
OF HIGH SCHOOL SENIORS

Choice	Black 1974		Black 1985		Coloured 1974		Coloured 1985		Indian 1974		Indian 1985		White 1974		White 1985	
	No.	%	No.	%	No.	%	No.	%	No.	%	No.	%	No.	%	No.	%
Anglican*	27	14.7			18	20.5			4	1.2			103	23.5		
Catholic	60	32.6	47	38.8	54	61.5	109	61.2	7	2.2	10	3.0	71	16.2	61	15.1
Dutch Reformed	7	3.8	3	2.5	2	2.2	1	0.6			4	1.2	65	14.8	63	15.6
Hindu									254	78.1	228	68.1			1	0.2
Muslim					6	6.8	10	5.6	47	14.4	36	10.7				
Methodist	43	23.3	37	30.6	2	2.2	3	1.7	3	0.9	8	2.4	91	20.7	116	28.8
Presbyterian	9	4.9	5	4.1			1	0.6	3	0.9	9	2.7	95	21.6	37	9.2
Episcopalian			2	1.7											2	0.5
Jewish											1	0.3			11	2.7
Shembe			2	1.7												
Other (includes separatists)	38	20.7	25	20.7	6	6.8	54	30.3	7	2.2	39	11.6	14	3.1	112	27.8
Total	184	100.0	121	100.0	88	100.0	178	100.0	325	99.9	335	100.0	439	99.9	403	100.0
No response			5				2				6				9	

* Through an oversight this category was deleted in the 1985 survey, *assuming* students would recognize its equivalence in the Episcopal church. This obviously did not occur.

51

In terms of participation in group worship, that is church attendance or related activities, we found that the Coloureds remained the most active. In 1974 some 69.7 percent indicated that they attended church on a weekly basis; in 1985 that figure was 61.5 percent. The attendance pattern for the other three groups also changed as the students indicated that church attendance among Blacks was 47.5 percent (35.1 percent in 1974), among Indians 37.1 percent (27.5 percent in 1974), and among Whites 32.2 percent (37.2 percent in 1974).

We should keep in mind that in 1974, 78.1 percent of the Indian students were Hindu, and a great deal of their religious ritual occurred in the home. When asked who attended worship services only on religious holy days, the Indians had the highest attendance rate (48.1 percent), the Whites (15.4 percent) and the Coloureds (6.7 percent). In 1985 we found that 68.1 percent of Indians were Hindu. The two major Indian religions had both lost members to Christian churches, particularly to pentecostalism. Again they were trailed by others in terms of students attending only on religious holy days: Indians (38.8 percent), Blacks (16.1 percent), Whites (13.1 percent) and Coloureds (10.1 percent).

Those who indicated that they did not attend church or religious gatherings at all, not even on religious holy days, remained constant except for an increase among the Whites. Among the Coloureds in both 1974 and 1985, only 5.6 percent indicated no religious activity. Among the Indians the figure was down slightly from 15.9 percent in 1974 to 15.5 percent in 1985; the Blacks more than doubled from 5.1 percent in 1974 to 12.0 percent in 1985. Whites who claimed to have had no formal religious activity decreased from 33.5 percent to 25.9 in 1985.

The Afrikaner has been described as very religious in the sense of denominational membership, church attendance, and participation in religious activities and festivities. The Afrikaans medium school is clearly distinguishable from the English medium schools in this study. Whereas the three English medium White schools, respectively, had 32.7 percent (girls' school), 44.4 percent (boys' school), and 39.7 percent (city outskirts) of the students who indicated that they did "not at all" attend services, only 12.3 percent of the students in the Afrikaans medium school were so involved. Not a single one of the latter school's students attended church only on religious holy days. As a group the Afrikaans students thus were more religiously active and involved than any of the other categories; the Coloureds were second.

Social clubs

Since we had a question in a later section of the questionnaire pertaining to incorporating a known cannabis smoker in a social club, we asked who belonged to such a club. Under clubs we included such organized activities as debating societies, athletic clubs, student Christian associations, and so forth. Nothing important emerged except that about half the students in each category belonged to associations.

Social clubs and student associations should be contrasted with sports clubs and activities. Unless the school makes provision for meeting times during school hours or breaks, activities are limited to after school hours. Since none of these schools have dormitories, students would have to remain after school or return in the afternoon or evening. For Black, Coloureds, and Indians this obviously involves particular problems regarding transportation and safety. In many cases, especially Blacks, students reside in badly lit areas or in ghettos without lighting.

Family background

A number of questions concentrated on the composition of the family in which the students were reared, the age at which changes such as death or divorce occurred that altered the family composition, and the emotional relationship felt by students toward their parents or guardians. These data were important to establish, for tensions, frustrations, or feelings of hostility frequently spill over into experimentation with or abuse of mind or mood altering substances.

Most students grew up in nuclear families where the father and mother were present. Blacks were the only group which showed an increase in this category. In 1974 some 59.6 percent of Black students grew up in a nuclear family setting; by 1985 this figure had risen to 65.9 percent. The change represents improved living conditions for Blacks. When the earlier study was conducted, Blacks lived under the shadow of possible eviction.

The Native Laws Amendment Act (No. 54 of 1952), particularly as it applied to urban Blacks, was one of the laws which affected Black residents. This law permitted a Black person born in South Africa to visit an urban area for up to seventy-two hours without requiring a special permit. In terms of influx control and referring specifically to Black women, it defined very clearly who may reside in urban areas. Authorities were given wide powers to order the removal of Blacks they considered to be "idle or undesirable." The law provided that no Black could remain in an urban or proclaimed area for more than seventy-two hours, unless he or she fulfilled one of the following conditions:

1. Had resided there continuously since birth
2. Had worked there continuously for one employer for not less than ten years or had resided there lawfully and continuously for not less than fifteen years and had thereafter continued to reside there and was not employed outside and had not during this time been sentenced to a fine exceeding R100 or to imprisonment for a period exceeding six months
3. Was the wife, unmarried daughter, or son under the age of eighteen years of a Black in one of the categories mentioned above and ordinarily resided with him
4. Had been granted special permission to be in the area

In 1964 an Amendment (Act No. 42) was passed which established that to qualify for section (3) above, the said person initially must have entered the area "lawfully"—usually defined in terms of length of residence and employment. The last amendment also, for the first time, allowed persons who qualified for urban residences under the previous four conditions to be deemed idle or undesirable and then to be ordered out of a prescribed area. The four conditions listed above are generally known as Section 10(1) and became the critical factors by which urban Blacks are measured.

Until 1964 qualification under Section 10(1) gave an urban Black a new lease on life. He could be allocated a home; he could find employment; he could have his family with him and go about his daily living with only minor fear of police interrogation. For many years such relative certainty and predictability did not exist, but with the lifting of restrictions on influx control since 1990, family life may become more normal for Black South Africans. Any spot check for passes, police raid, or labor unrest immediately led officials to weigh the person against Section 10(1) and then to evaluate exactly how 'idle or undesirable' he was. In talking with urban Blacks one was repeatedly struck by their fear of officialdom and the tenuousness of their existence in the city. The very worst possible punishment for a sophisticated urban resident was to be returned to the intellectual barrenness and poverty of his homeland.

The certainty and predictability of urban residence was further shattered in January 1968 when a directive issued by the Department of Bantu Administration and Development decreed that Blacks living in urban areas no longer were permitted to build their own houses on their thirty-year leasehold plots. They could neither buy nor inherit such homes. Many had paid in cash for their homes in order that their children or widows would have the certainty of homes; others had made initial cash down payments and were paying monthly amounts toward purchase of their houses. The decree stated that those urban Blacks who already had purchased their houses might dispose of them only to the local urban authority concerned. Houses which had been purchased could not be bequeathed to their heirs. Tenants who had improved their homes by adding rooms, laying on water, building a porch, or some other alteration, would not be compensated for these improvements when the tenants left. Further, Government Notice R.1036 of June 1968 made it clear that family housing permits could be issued only to South African Black males who were over twenty-one years old and who qualified in terms of Section 10(1) (a) or (b) of the Urban Areas Act to remain in the city, who were lawfully employed there and who had dependents legally living with them. Thus a Black widower, a widow, someone with a special permit, who lost his job and was unemployed for thirty days, who became divorced or who went on pension automatically qualified for removal from the urban area.

By 1985, due to relaxation of enforcement and new laws, predictability about residence had improved significantly and a greater deal of security was experienced. However, Blacks still had the lowest percentage of students who were residing with both mother and father. Coloured students came from similar homes; only 66.1 percent were from homes where both parents were present. These two ethnic groups also showed the highest percentage of students who lived with a divorced parent. In spite of this slight rise which may represent better living conditions, we should also take note of marital changes which had taken place in South Africa. Specifically, this was a sociological phenomenon which should be seen against a growing trend in southern Africa in which female-headed households were becoming very common. Among Indian (82.7 percent) and White (85.0 percent) students there was a larger percentage who resided in the nuclear family with both parents. In those cases where a smaller number of students grew up in a nuclear family setting, we are dealing not only with higher rates of divorce or separation but also with widowhood.

Asked about their relationship with a parent or guardian, most students indicated "very good." Black students were the highest at 94.2 percent (up from 92.0 percent in 1974), while Coloured students were the lowest at 89.5 percent (down from 96.3 percent in 1974). This represents normal domestic relations with close to warm relationship between parents and off-spring.

Socio-economic factors

The picture regarding job type (which also reflects on social status, security, and long term prospects) and level of income emerged from the questions posed in 1974. Because of the length of the survey questionnaire and the time involved, questions asking students to describe the occupation of the main provider in their family and to estimate the total income of the family were not repeated in 1985.

In 1974, as was expected, these questions produced the greatest contrasts between different ethnic categories and highlighted socio-economic differences which were based on color and group membership. Our first question concerned the occupation of the household head. The range of possibilities is too extensive for all to be reproduced here. The greatest variation occurred among White and Indian parents, while Black parents had the least range of alternatives. Whites showed the largest percentage of managerial (10.8 percent) and professional (17.5

percent) parents; Blacks showed the lowest percentages in these categories. The highest percentage of domestic servant and laborer types, as well as 12.3 percent who were listed as teachers, also occurred among Black subjects.

When one translated job type to income, much the same picture emerged but in sharper detail. Only 1.0 percent of White, 19.5 percent of Coloured, and 19.8 percent of Indian pupils indicated that their parents earned less than *R90 per month* or *R1080 per year*; 69.7 percent of Black pupils indicated this income level for the parent or breadwinner. At the other end of the income scale we find only one Black pupil indicating that his parents earned more than *R530 per month* or *R6360 per year*, whereas 2.1 percent of Indian, 5.6 percent of Coloured and an impressive 40.6 percent of White pupils' parents earned that amount.[1]

Whites quite obviously were in a favorable and enviable position in terms of a wide range of job choices and dependable income which guaranteed family security. Indians also had a range of job possibilities but less security owing to lower income as was the case with the Coloureds. Black South Africans were in the sad state of being controlled in terms of residence rights, restricted in terms of job reservations, and also of being less educated, having fewer job skills, and receiving lower wages overall. It should also be recalled that most of the low paying jobs had no social security or pension privileges. These facts must be reflected in the attitudes and aims of students and are no doubt connected to the expression of future plans discussed above.

In the intervening decade some significant changes had taken place in South Africa. Salaries had increased (but so had the cost of living), hotels and restaurants were integrated (but this hardly benefitted a family living near the poverty line), universities were now "open" (little comfort to the uneducated laborer or semi-skilled worker). Overall, it would seem, the relative position and condition of the various ethnic groups had remained the same. In 1985 Whites still had a favorable status, still had the greatest range

---

[1]Though the values of the South African Rand and the U.S. dollar fluctuate in relation to each other, there was an approximate equivalency in 1978 of one U.S. dollar to one South African Rand.

of jobs as well as possible job mobility, and their incomes still were higher and more secure than that of the other ethnic groups. Blacks were still running last and reaching for advantages.

Settlement patterns

Rounding out general background information on students in the school sample, a question asked, "Where did you live during most of the past six years?" The reason for this question was that since most of the students were about seventeen or eighteen years of age, the answer would establish where they had spent the greater part of their teenage years and also suggest the kind of influences to which they had been exposed.

Responses indicated that in 1985 as in 1974 we were dealing with essentially an urban community. Figures show that students in the twelve high schools under study had an even greater urban base than before. This suggests that a smaller number of families were recent urban immigrants or that a larger number of families had spent most of their children's teenage years in the city.

In spite of the original Indian indentured laborers having come to reside in rural areas as agricultural workers, their children and grandchildren became urban migrants, taking jobs in cities, establishing trade stores on city outskirts, or farming small tracts where fruit and vegetables were produced. In time the Indian population became essentially an urban population. This was also reflected in the figures for residence of students. While 91.3 percent of the 1974 sample had spent most of their lives in the city, 97.7 percent of the 1985 sample had done so.

Coloureds in Natal, as contrasted with those in the Cape, formed a relatively small and select group who were better educated and urban in residence. This population lacked the characteristics of rural unskilled farm workers so typical of Coloureds living in small towns or engaged in fruit and viniculture in the Western Cape Province. Urban characteristics were reflected in the fact that urban residence of Coloured students increased from 94.3 percent in 1974 to 97.2 percent in 1985.

The most spectacular change was reflected in the residence of White students. In the first study, 79.7 percent of the high school seniors had spent their teen years in a city; but by 1985, the percentage had risen to 93.7. This increase suggests the stabilization of an urban population with fewer rural migrants, fewer farmers settling in the city, and therefore, a more prolonged urban influence on young people during their formative years.

The last of the four population groups is the only one with an authentic rural home base in the form of traditional residence patterns and integrated social system. Black students recognize this tradition. In many cases rural linkages and networks are retained and cultivated as personnel and goods flow in both directions. In 1974 only 81.1 percent of the Black students had spent most of their youth years in a city and by 1985 this figure had risen only slightly to 83.0 percent. Based on extensive research, this writer can suggest that a fairly large number of Black students were familiar with traditional cultural values, institutions, and lifestyle. This would include the traditional value of cannabis and methods of its use, information readily shared with peer group members in the segregated residential areas which mark South African demographics.

Because most of the students in both samples had spent the greater part of their teen years, indeed of their lives, in a city, they had been exposed to urban influences, including a variety of drugs, certain ways of acquiring drugs, and patterns as well as places associated with the use of drugs. In 1985, as had been the case a decade earlier, "drugs" referred essentially to alcohol and cannabis.

Summary

The material presented in this chapter gives a thumbnail sketch of the South African society. It has illuminated the social and demographic background of high school seniors. It has placed them in ethnically separate communities regulated by the Group Areas Act with multiple amendments, and it has highlighted the favorable conditions of Whites. Any society develops proper and expected conditions and sequences. When people or groups do not operate according to expectations or meet the sequencing, they are on the margin of the wider society.

One societal expectation in South Africa was that a child goes to school at age six and by eighteen should be a senior. If a grade had to be repeated or if illness resulted in long absences, such a student might not be "on time." Among White students, 90 percent were seniors at age seventeen or eighteen; among Indians 86 percent are; 78 percent of Coloured seniors usually graduated high school on time. Not only were Blacks behind the schedule with only 21 percent in this age classification, but they also showed the greatest range of age. Seniors were positioned on an age range from sixteen to over twenty-three. The reasons for this disparity were multiple and complex, but all reflected on the second-class citizenship of Blacks and the inferiority of conditions—at home, in the townships, and at school. A person cannot be "on time" if everything else is delaying him.

There never has been preference for schooling among people in South Africa as regards gender or birth order. Once primary and perhaps secondary school has been completed, it frequently was the son in a family who was permitted and supported into tertiary and professional education. Depending on the family and at what stage needs or crises arise, this may also result in the eldest or the youngest being given a chance at furthering his or her education. In the case of Indian South Africans, however, there was a very clear pattern of girls being withdrawn from school upon reaching menarche. This is discussed fully and in context in du Toit's (1990) study of aging and menopause among Indian South African women. The situation started to change some years ago, and in the latest study reported on here, Indian girls in the senior class were almost equal in numbers to boys. This represented a clear increase over the numbers of a decade earlier.

As to language, there was a clear movement toward English as the most frequently used language. We found traditional Indian languages being replaced by English among Indian students, African languages gradually being replaced among Blacks, and Afrikaans being replaced among the Coloured students. This was in keeping with the South African constitution in which English and Afrikaans are both official languages, and school instruction must include both. The Afrikaans medium school for Whites thus would teach English but remain a linguistic enclave in Durban.

The conditions resulting in the grade age discrepancy and the situation created by that discrepancy had a clear effect on the future plans of high school seniors. To a certain extent "future plans" contained a wish list—they were the ideals, dreams, and hopes which a person has at that time. Economic conditions, however, enter as a test of reality. We found that to improve themselves and to get away from low pay and poor socioeconomic conditions, the greater majority of Black seniors would have liked to have gone to college. Translated into the South African idiom, this implied either university (to study for a degree which could be used for teaching) or teachers' training college. Both implied a steady salary and prestige.

Religious group membership does not imply religiosity, and religiosity does not guarantee a drug free lifestyle. But it has been found time and time again that religiosity does result in a social milieu and friendship networks which are less likely to include drug use and drug users. Our findings confirmed that while White students had become less religious in the last decade, Afrikaans students were the most religious, in terms of membership and participation, of all the sub-categories.

Finally, in terms of family composition, we found a contradiction in the social versus the legal position of Blacks. Nationwide in South Africa, Blacks were moving toward woman-headed households. The reasons for this trend were complex and cannot be discussed here, but women were taking the initiative. This does not imply not having a family. Rose Modise, a factory worker featured in a study, *Working Women*, explained as follows:

> A lot of women don't get married these days—especially in Soweto. I've got a friend who's a social worker. She's got a baby and says she doesn't want to get married. The father wants to marry, but she won't.
>
> I don't want my daughters to get married. If they are educated it's better that they earn a living wage. Marriage, I don't care for it. I'd like them to stay with me. They can have children and support them. They will have a better life. In Soweto marriage is no more.
>
> I think it's caused by drinking. Men drink too much after they get married. The wife looks and thinks, "No, I can do without." Women bring the money in and men stay at home because they don't want to work. Some men are already crippled by liquor. So he's just an extra baby for the wife. He wants money for smokes and beer. She has to buy him clothes and feed him like a baby.

Women have just decided not to get married. Some are divorced—there are plenty of divorcees who won't get married again. They're tired of it. Soon there will be no more marriage. Just boyfriends and girlfriends. (Sached 1985:11)

This attitude towards marriage conflicts with the requirements of housing in government-run townships. Housing is based on marriage and employment. As there have been in the past, so in the future there will be many ways of circumventing officialdom.

4

STUDENT USE OF CANNABIS AND ALCOHOL

Introduction

What is use? How often should a person use drugs to be classified as a user? In the 1974 drug survey we followed the accepted criteria and had no reason to change it in the most recent study. In agreement with Keniston (1968) and Greenwald and Leutgert (1971), we adopted the prevailing definition of "drug user" as anyone who has ever tried any one of the consciousness altering substances. Stated differently, any person who has used an illegal drug removed himself from the category of non-users and has been designated a user, with potentially vast social, interactional, and behavioral implications (du Toit 1976a). The next entry on our questionnaire was critical in that it asked about the student's use of cannabis. Because the students were working in complete privacy, without a teacher in attendance, and with my assurance of complete anonymity, we accepted the results as a true and honest reflection of the drug use pattern in the schools under consideration.

History of student cannabis use

The first part of the survey questionnaire on drug use dealt with student's family background and the social person. In the second part, we turned specifically to the use of cannabis and the students were clearly so informed. The first question was phrased "During your life-time, have you used dagga?" The answer allowed for different expressions of frequency ranging from "never" to "twenty or more times." Respondents giving the latter answer we counted as regular users. Table 5 reflects this information.

Table 5

HISTORY OF CANNABIS USE BY HIGH SCHOOL SENIORS

Frequency	Black				Coloured				Indian				White			
	1974		1985		1974		1985		1974		1985		1974		1985	
	No.	%	No.	%	No.	%	No.	%	No.	%	No.	%	No.	%	No.	%
Never	188	82.8	118	93.7	78	87.6	146	81.1	269	80.1	273	80.1	425	85.7	337	81.8
Once or twice	19	8.4	2	1.6	5	5.7	16	8.9	30	8.9	43	12.6	27	5.5	41	10.0
3-5 times	6	2.7	1	0.8	3	3.4	6	3.3	8	2.3	9	2.6	14	2.9	14	3.4
6-9 times	0	0.0	0	0.0	1	1.1	2	1.1	7	2.1	6	1.8	7	1.4	3	0.7
10-14 times	3	1.3	0	0.0	0	0.0	1	0.6	2	0.6	3	0.9	2	0.2	2	0.5
15-19 times	1	0.4	0	0.0	0	0.0	1	0.6	2	0.6	1	0.3	4	0.8	1	0.2
20+	10	4.4	5	4.0	2	2.2	8	4.4	18	5.4	6	1.8	17	3.5	14	3.4
Total	227	100.0	126	100.0	89	100.0	180	100.0	336	100.0	341	100.0	496	100.0	412	100.0
No response	1								1				2			

64

In comparing the history of cannabis use by high school seniors, it is interesting to note two salient features. The Black students not only have the highest percentage who claim never to have used this drug, but they are also the only group for whom this category has increased. (Note that the category "never used" differs slightly between Table 5 and Table 6.) However, while Blacks claim the largest percentage who have never used, they share with Coloured students the highest percentage who claim to have used the drug twenty times or more. Based on these figures one might venture that Black students either do not use cannabis at all, or use it on a regular basis. Given the tradition of cannabis use among the indigenous Africans, we might have expected and did find regular users who justify the practice on the basis that it is an African tradition or that it is a part of their culture. These figures of use contrast with the other three student groups among whom there are respondents who claim a variety of patterns of use.

In 1985, among Coloured, Indian, and White students almost 19 percent claimed to have used cannabis at various intervals. For the Coloureds and Whites this percentage was up from the figures in 1974; among Coloured from 12.4 percent to 18.9 percent and among White students from 14.3 percent to 18.2 percent. For the Indians it was identical: 20.0 percent.

People who use drugs include those who experiment as well as those who are regular users. Since we were dealing here with young people, it was even more important to differentiate between regular users and those who experimented or tried a drug under peer group pressure or while trying to impress friends and who most likely would not repeat the action. The descriptions we were given in the ethnographic study indicated that "first use" or "first trip" frequently was not very pleasant. Experimenters ranged from the young fellow in the village who had to clean his grandfather's cannabis pipe (yes, he went behind the shed and tried it out!) to the youth who joined friends in the urban setting in smoking a *zol* or cannabis cigarette.

If students indicated that they had used cannabis, they were requested to indicate frequency in response to the question concerning the last time they had used this drug. These figures essentially confirmed the finding represented in Table 5, that those

65

who indicated they used twenty times or more were also the same students who claim to have used cannabis during the last week.

During the same time frame (1973-1974), van der Burgh administered a study questionnaire to a total of 4,588 White males, aged sixteen to twenty-one. The researchers were interested in both cannabis and other (illicit) drug use. The findings were that 20.1 percent of the total sample had used cannabis and other drugs; but only 15.4 percent had used cannabis only. The author explained: "Of those admitting drug use, 708 (76.7 percent) reported having used only dagga at least once, 202 (21.9 percent) had used both dagga and other drugs at least once while 13 (1.4 percent) had used only other drugs at least once" (van der Burgh 1975:10). The largest percentage of these persons was composed of experimental and occasional users.

Frequency of student drug use

Of generally greater significance was the next question which asked how frequently each student smoked cannabis. The results are presented in Table 6. These figures agree to a major extent with the previous discussion and indicate that their actual frequency of use was very close to their perceived frequency. (There is a slight variance between those who previously had claimed never to have used and those who in 1985 stated that they had never used.)

According to the information supplied in this table, only 5.6 percent of the Black students used cannabis in 1985, down from 14.9 percent in 1974. Among the other groups the figures were respectively 17.2 percent (up from 12.2 percent) for the Coloureds; 17.3 percent (up from 15.6 percent) for the Indians; and 16.5 percent (up from 13.3 percent) for the Whites. It is instructive to compare these figures with those of other countries. In 1984 40 percent of United States high school students reported using marijuana (Johnston and O'Malley 1986). In Australia, one study (Campion et al. 1978) reported 62 percent of the students using cannabis. In a survey conducted in 1977 (Kandel 1981) only three percent of Israeli youths reported having ever tried cannabis. Anumonye (1980), using a sample of 2,846 pupils from seventeen secondary schools in Nigeria, found that 2.9 percent of the males and 2.1 percent of the females used cannabis. Other studies

Table 6

FREQUENCY OF CANNABIS USE BY HIGH SCHOOL SENIORS

Frequency	Black				Coloured				Indian				White			
	1974		1985		1974		1985		1974		1985		1974		1985	
	No.	%	No.	%	No.	%	No.	%	No.	%	No.	%	No.	%	No.	%
Never	189	85.1	119	94.4	78	87.8	149	82.8	270	84.4	282	82.7	418	86.7	344	83.5
Daily or more	5	2.3	4	3.2	0	0.0	2	1.1	7	2.2	2	0.6	3	0.6	2	0.5
Once week or more	12	5.4	1	0.8	2	2.2	4	2.2	5	1.6	9	2.6	10	2.1	5	1.2
1-3 times a month	2	0.9	0	0.0	0	0.0	1	0.6	7	2.2	2	0.6	10	2.1	8	1.9
Every 2-3 months	1	0.5	0	0.0	2	2.2	2	1.1	6	1.9	3	0.9	9	1.9	7	1.7
2-3 times a year	0	0.0	1	0.8	2	2.2	7	3.9	11	3.4	10	2.9	13	2.7	14	3.4
Once a year or less	13	5.9	1	0.8	5	5.6	15	8.4	14	4.4	33	9.7	19	3.9	32	7.8
Total	222	100.0	126	100.0	89	100.0	180	100.0	320	100.0	341	100.0	482	100.0	412	100.0
No response	6								17				16			

(Nevadomsky 1981) support the finding that cannabis use among West African students was not prevalent.

But what about White students? We do know that this group occupied the most favorable status in a socioeconomic sense and that they not only had more money but also more leisure time than the other groups. In contrast to the other groups, White South Africans permitted a contrast between an English speaking population being generally more secular and having more international cultural contacts than the Afrikaans speaking population. On the whole the latter were more traditionally conservative, religious, and culturally isolationist.

If we look in some detail at the White sample from Durban, we find that cannabis use was more prevalent among English speaking pupils. It was also more prevalent among males. Thus, if we compare the Whites who had ever used cannabis, Table 7 shows that the English medium co-educational school more closely resembles the other English medium schools and these three contrast quite sharply with the Afrikaans medium school in Durban. The school with greatest drug use was the boys' high school, where in 1974 22.0 percent claimed that they used cannabis. By 1985 this figure was up to 36.6 percent. The girls' school also shows an increase from 10.6 percent in 1974 to 13.1 percent a decade later and matched the co-educational institutions which actually showed a decline from 13.9 percent to 12.9 percent. In contrast and in spite of a 100 percent increase of those who claimed to have used cannabis (the Afrikaans medium school showed an increase from 2.4 percent to 4.9 percent in the eleven years under review) the Afrikaans medium school still had the lowest percentage of users. The two schools in the wealthy, prestigious neighborhood showed not only higher percentages of use but a higher percentage of use especially among the males, figures which compare well with those for the United States and Europe.

It is interesting to compare these same schools on the use of alcohol, a subject not covered in the 1974 survey. The first question in a section dealing with the use of alcohol allowed students to indicate frequency of use. Once again we found that only 10.5 percent of the students at the Afrikaans medium high school indicated weekly (or more frequent) use of alcohol (Table 8). All the other schools had figures at least double that frequency

Table 7

FREQUENCY OF CANNABIS USE BY WHITE HIGH SCHOOL SENIORS

| | English Medium High School on City Outskirts | | | | Afrikaans Medium Urban High School | | | | English Medium Wealthy Neighborhood Boys School | | | | English Medium Wealthy Neighborhood Girls School | | | |
| | 1974 | | 1985 | | 1974 | | 1985 | | 1974 | | 1985 | | 1974 | | 1985 | |
Frequency	No.	%	No.	%	No.	%	No.	%	No.	%	No.	%	No.	%	No.	%
Never	99	86.1	115	87.1	82	97.6	78	95.1	110	78.0	57	63.3	127	89.4	94	87.0
Daily or more	1	0.9	1	0.8	1	1.2	1	1.2	2	1.4	0	0.0	1	0.7	0	0.0
Once week or more	1	0.9	4	3.0	1	1.2	0	0.0	7	5.0	1	1.1	0	0.0	0	0.0
1-3 times a month	2	1.7	2	1.5	0	0.0	0	0.0	3	2.1	4	4.4	5	3.5	2	1.9
Every 2-3 months	4	3.5	1	0.8	0	0.0	0	0.0	4	2.8	4	4.4	1	0.7	2	1.9
2-3 times a year	3	2.6	5	3.8	0	0.0	0	0.0	8	5.7	6	6.7	2	1.4	3	2.8
Once a year or less	5	4.3	4	3.0	0	0.0	3	3.7	7	5.0	18	20.0	6	4.2	7	6.5
Total	115	100.0	132	100.0	84	100.0	82	100.0	141	100.0	90	99.9	142	100.0	108	100.1
No response	4				4				5				3			

Table 8

FREQUENCY OF ALCOHOL USE BY WHITE HIGH
SCHOOL SENIORS IN 1985

Frequency	English Medium High School on City Outskirts		Afrikaans Medium Urban High School		English Medium Wealthy Neighborhood Boys School		English Medium Wealthy Neighborhood Girls School	
	Number	Percent	Number	Percent	Number	Percent	Number	Percent
Daily or more	3	2.5	-	-	2	2.2	-	-
Once week or more	34	28.1	8	10.5	38	42.7	21	20.0
1-3 times a month	37	30.6	22	28.9	27	30.3	39	37.1
2-3 times a month	21	17.4	20	26.3	9	10.1	20	19.0
2-3 times a year	15	12.4	13	17.1	8	9.0	14	13.3
Once a year or less	11	9.1	13	17.1	5	5.6	11	10.5
Total	·121	100.1	76	99.9	89	99.9	105	99.9
No response	11		6		1		3	

with almost half the students in the boys' school indicating this frequency.

Let us, however, return to the subject of cannabis use and specifically to attitudes about this drug. There are, of course, a number of persons who use cannabis once or even a number of times and then stop. Some of these people may simply have been experimenting, others reacting to situational peer pressure, and still others may have had a bad experience or perhaps may have arrived at a logical reason for discontinuing its use. On the questionnaire the two logical reasons most frequently indicated by students were "physical and mental risk" of smoking cannabis, and especially the "legal risk" of using an illegal drug. It could be suggested that the latter would serve as a deterrent in a country with very stringent drug laws, strict enforcement, and a rigid caste system which was showing signs of weakening and permitting upward mobility of minority group members.*

The question of future use is related to the reasons for discontinuing use (or never having used). In their study of Chilean students, Comberoff and his associates (1972:28) found that among nonsmokers, 17.3 percent were ready to smoke cannabis in future. As indicated in Table 9, the students in our sample showed approximately the same distribution, with the highest frequency among Whites. This group also showed the greatest change of those who intend to use; 5.6 percent more in 1985 than in 1974. Black and Indian students showed a clear decline in total percentages of those who expected to use this drug. The most dramatic change occurred among Indian students. Those students who were quite sure that they would smoke cannabis and intended to use it on a regular basis came from the Black and White groups. The former has the longest tradition of use; the latter the greatest socioeconomic ability for drug acquisition.

In a study of drug use among American high school seniors (du Toit 1978; du Toit and Suggs 1983), we discerned a disturbing trend toward an increasing number of students who had their first drug experience before or in middle school. This meant that by

---

*See du Toit (1966) for a discussion of the dynamics of a color-caste system as it changes into a system of classes based on color.

71

Table 9

EXPECTED USE OF CANNABIS DURING THE NEXT YEAR
BY HIGH SCHOOL SENIORS

Frequency	Black 1974		Black 1985		Coloured 1974		Coloured 1985		Indian 1974		Indian 1985		White 1974		White 1985	
	No.	%	No.	%	No.	%	No.	%	No.	%	No.	%	No.	%	No.	%
More than once or twice	6	2.7	6	4.9	2	2.2	1	0.6	12	3.6	2	0.6	8	1.6	10	2.4
No more than once or twice	1	0.5	2	1.6	0	0.0	3	1.7	5	1.5	4	1.2	8	1.6	7	1.7
Maybe once or twice	8	3.5	1	0.8	5	5.6	9	5.1	18	5.5	17	5.1	19	3.6	28	6.8
Probably not	20	9.0	5	4.1	3	3.4	9	5.1	22	6.6	10	3.0	50	10.2	48	11.7
Definitely not	187	84.2	109	88.6	79	88.8	154	87.5	272	83.0	299	90.1	407	82.9	317	77.3
Total	222	100.0	123	100.0	89	100.0	176	100.0	329	100.0	332	100.0	492	100.0	410	100.0
No response	6		3				4		8		9		6		2	

the time these students entered high school (grades nine through twelve), many had already acquired the habit or at least experimented with drugs. The equivalent age and grade level in the South African system would be standard seven through ten. High school in South Africa, however, starts with standard six (more or less age thirteen).

Questioned in 1974 about their first use of cannabis, the students indicated that their initial introduction to the drug occurred during high school. Twice as many Indian and Coloured students had started in standard nine or ten, that is within the previous two years before being questioned. This was not as clear in the case of White and Black students. Table 10 shows that a small number of Black, Indians, and Whites were introduced to and started smoking cannabis before they went to high school. During the first three years in high school, however, more than twice as many Blacks started smoking as did their age-mates who started some years later. The 10.5 percent who started in junior high (standard six through eight) was the highest single total and pointed to a younger starting age of cannabis smokers among Blacks. An extenuating fact which normally applies in these comparative discussions does show up here—the relatively older overall age of Blacks in school. The 3.2 percent of young (sixteen-year-old) Black students in their final year of high school in 1985, compared well with the other groups: White 3.6 percent, Coloured 2.8 percent, and Indian 0.3 percent. But the other end of the age continuum is clearly skewed. Those students who were nineteen years and older in their senior year represented only 5.8 percent of the Whites, 13.2 percent of the Indians, and 19.5 percent of the Coloureds. Among Black students this older category represented 76.0 percent of the student population covered by this study.[*] We can state then, with a great degree of empirical support, that Black students in high school are not only older but normally have a great deal more "street wisdom" about drugs because of having grown up in racial ghettos outside South African cities.

---

[*]For comparable figures among girls in two Black schools in Pretoria, see du Toit (1987).

Table 10

HISTORY OF FIRST CANNABIS USE
BY HIGH SCHOOL SENIORS

Time Period	Black				Coloured				Indian				White			
	1974		1985		1974		1985		1974		1985		1974		1985	
	No.	%	No.	%	No.	%	No.	%	No.	%	No.	%	No.	%	No.	%
Never Used	188	82.5	117	92.9	78	87.6	146	81.1	267	79.2	275	80.7	425	85.7	337	81.8
Prior to high school	5	2.2	1	0.8	0	0.0	1	0.6	4	1.2	3	0.9	3	0.6	4	1.0
During STD 6-8	24	10.5	6	4.8	3	3.4	13	7.2	21	6.2	24	7.0	31	6.3	31	7.5
During STD 9-10	11	4.8	2	1.6	8	9.0	20	11.1	45	13.4	39	11.4	37	7.5	40	9.7
Total	228	100.0	126	100.0	89	100.0	180	100.0	337	100.0	341	100.0	496	100.0	412	100.0
No response															2	

From data in the 1985 questionnaire about first use of cannabis, we see in Table 9 that about 41.0 percent of Coloured, Indians, and Whites who had smoked cannabis started this drug use prior to their two senior years of high school, compared to 77.7 percent of the Black student users who did. Nevertheless, this figure dropped significantly between 1974, when 12.7 percent of all Black students started prior to their senior years, to 1985 when only 5.6 percent did so.

The social background

The age of first use may be determined largely by social relationships. Table 11 shows that among the students in all four categories, neighborhood friends and school friends were the primary agents of introduction. Kinsmen, appearing under "other," figure very slightly except among the Coloured. In the Black sample families were relatively large, but traditions of use usually excluded an older person participating with one younger than himself.

This would imply that schoolmates, or at least persons in the same age category, were the most frequent smoking companions. From our total sample of the four ethnic groups, only two persons indicated that they smoked exclusively at school; eight persons stated that they sometimes smoked at school. These ten persons form a very small number in our total sample of 193 smokers.

Significant changes occurred from 1974 to 1985 in relation to the influence of friends at school on smoking habits in both the Black and White groups. In the Black group, responses to whether friends at school influenced the respondent to smoke cannabis dropped from 5.3 percent in 1974 to 0.8 percent in 1985. The opposite trend was evident among White students: those being influenced by their school peers to smoke cannabis rose from 3.9 percent in 1974 to 6.1 percent in 1985. We find that the reverse is true regarding neighborhood friends: there is a significant drop in influence among Black students, a relatively stable influence among Indian and White, and a clear increase in influence among Coloured drug users. The importance of the peer group has been discussed by Bruce Johnson. He wrote "that persons who spend a great deal of time with their peer group in relative isolation from adult controls are likely to engage in a wide variety of uncon-

Table 11

WHO INTRODUCED THE STUDENT TO CANNABIS USE?

Who Introduced?	Black				Coloured				Indian				White			
	1974		1985		1974		1985		1974		1985		1974		1985	
	No.	%	No.	%	No.	%	No.	%	No.	%	No.	%	No.	%	No.	%
Never Used	186	81.6	116	92.1	78	87.6	147	81.7	267	79.5	272	79.8	422	85.3	336	81.6
Neighborhood friends	19	8.3	3	2.4	5	5.6	18	10.0	39	11.6	41	12.0	36	7.6	32	7.8
Friends in other city	5	2.2	2	1.6	1	1.1	3	1.7	5	1.5	2	0.6	4	0.8	8	1.9
Friends in rural area	3	1.3	1	0.8	0	0.0	3	1.7	3	0.9	4	1.2	6	1.2	2	0.5
Friends at school	12	5.3	1	0.8	2	2.2	7	3.9	16	4.7	18	5.3	19	3.9	25	6.1
Other	3	1.3	3	2.4	3	3.4	2	1.1	6	1.8	4	1.2	6	1.2	9	2.2
Total	228	100.0	126	100.0	89	100.0	180	100.0	336	100.0	341	100.0	493	100.0	412	100.0
No response									1				5			

ventional behaviour. In other words, the greater the peer cultural involvement, the greater the involvement in unconventional behaviour" (1973:7). When both parents work or when a child grows up in a single parent household, it is likely that proportionately more time will be spent in the company of peer group members.

If peers who are frequently neighborhood and school friends use cannabis, it is likely that students would count fellow cannabis smokers among their best friends at school. To test this conclusion we asked students "Of the three people you consider your best friends at school, how many have used dagga?" The emphasis then was on schoolmates and best friends in that context. The question was also specific and did not ask how many they think might have tried cannabis. But since we found earlier that neighborhood friends were very important, the same question was asked but substituted "at home" for "at school." In this way we could contrast school friends and neighborhood friends with the clear realization that these two categories may overlap considerably. Tables 12 and 13 present the results of these friendship questions.

Looking at the 1974 figures, it is obvious that a larger number of home friends than school friends smoke cannabis, and this is true for all the ethnic groups except the Indians. While Indians and Whites showed about the same percentage of school-using friends, the Whites had the highest percentage of home friends who smoke cannabis.

In the 1985 figures much the same pattern can be observed. Blacks claim to have had the fewest friends, at home or school, who smoked cannabis. In both studies Whites had maintained almost an identical pattern of home and school friends who used this drug. Two interesting phenomena can also be observed: first, the percentage who had no friends who used is lower in all cases than the percentage of nonusers in each ethnic category. Second, those students who had friends who used were always the highest percentage with one such friend and the lowest percentage of those who have three best friends who smoke cannabis. This suggests that we do not have a major case of social clustering of drug users. Alcohol use normally does not occur with a few select friends but at parties where most people will be using alcohol.

77

Table 12
NUMBER OF BEST FRIENDS AT SCHOOL
WHO USE CANNABIS

Number Who Use	Black				Coloured				Indian				White			
	1974		1985		1974		1985		1974		1985		1974		1985	
	No.	%	No.	%	No.	%	No.	%	No.	%	No.	%	No.	%	No.	%
None	164	72.2	103	81.7	71	79.8	129	71.7	240	71.2	248	72.7	352	71.0	291	70.6
One	11	4.8	5	4.0	9	10.1	20	11.1	36	10.7	33	9.7	65	13.1	47	11.4
Two	16	7.0	3	2.4	4	4.5	10	5.6	23	6.8	20	5.9	26	5.2	26	6.3
Three	7	3.1	4	3.2	0	0.0	6	3.3	17	5.0	17	5.0	23	4.6	14	3.4
Don't know	29	12.8	11	8.7	5	5.6	15	8.3	21	6.2	23	6.7	30	6.0	34	8.3
Total	227	100.0	126	100.0	89	100.0	180	100.0	337	100.0	341	100.0	496	100.0	412	100.0
No response	1												2			

Table 13
NUMBER OF BEST FRIENDS AT HOME
WHO USE CANNABIS

Number Who Use	Black				Coloured				Indian				White			
	1974		1985		1974		1985		1974		1985		1974		1985	
	No.	%	No.	%	No.	%	No.	%	No.	%	No.	%	No.	%	No.	%
None	144	63.5	99	78.6	63	70.8	126	70.0	251	75.4	219	64.2	334	67.3	298	72.3
One	22	9.6	6	4.8	13	14.6	19	10.6	32	9.6	49	14.4	71	14.3	48	11.7
Two	11	4.8	6	4.8	5	5.6	13	7.2	15	4.5	20	5.9	35	7.1	25	6.1
Three	13	5.7	4	3.2	3	3.4	14	7.8	18	5.4	23	6.7	29	5.8	16	3.9
Don't know	37	16.3	11	8.7	5	5.6	8	4.4	17	5.1	30	8.8	27	5.4	25	6.1
Total	227	100.0	126	100.0	89	100.0	180	100.0	333	100.0	341	100.0	496	100.0	412	100.0
No response	1								4				2			

When we turn our attention to alcohol use and friendship networks with persons known to use alcohol, the picture obtained from cannabis is reversed. Not only were there higher numbers, thus a greater percentage of friends who used alcohol, but those persons who had only one best friend who used alcohol were always smaller in number than those who have three best friends who used alcohol. This might suggest a greater clustering of alcohol users, but it most likely reflects the greater number of persons who use this "socially sanctioned" or legal drug and greater openness in its use.

This last point becomes clear if we look at the White students for whom these relationships were magnified. Students at the (White) boys' school show the clearest pattern: only 1.1 percent claim to have one best friend at home who drinks, but 82.8 percent claim three best friends who do. These figures are matched by the (White) girls' school as almost identical percentages appear. These two schools contrast sharply with the Afrikaans school where 19.4 percent claim to have only one best friend who drinks and only 48.6 percent who claim that all three of best friends use alcohol.

The final set of questions which dealt with the social background of the students in the research sample pertained to "significant others." The students were asked to indicate which person or group of persons they tried to please, either as persons or as students. The first question in this sequence asked them to rank the three persons or groups of people whose evaluation of them *as a person* concerned them most. The results were extremely interesting, particularly as regards Black versus White students. In 1974, some 60.5 percent of Black students indicated their parents were the most important, while only 48.5 percent of Whites made this selection. A decade later the same question was asked, and 94.2 percent of the Blacks and 77.9 percent of the Whites selected their parents. Coloured and Indian students on both surveys were in intermediate positions. The greatest single category in either of the two surveys was Black students singling out their mothers in 51.2 percent of their choices; Indians split evenly on mother and father, and Whites (all except the Afrikaans students) gave greater value to the opinion of the father.

The second most important category of "significant others" pertaining to these young people as "persons" follows a clear pattern. Black (31.3 percent) and Indian (22.6 percent) students select kinsmen, including siblings, uncles, aunts, and grandparents as the second most important group. This was true in 1974 and was confirmed in the 1985 survey. In contrast White and Coloured students selected friends, particularly boyfriend and girlfriend. In 1974 only 4.5 percent of Blacks indicated this category, and in 1985 only one student selected a girlfriend; in this same year among Indians, only 4.4 percent selected friends. However, among White students, 11.4 percent (down from 29.4 percent) selected friends as their second most important category; Coloureds made the same choice in 7.9 percent of the cases.

A detailed analysis of the White sample indicates that the Afrikaans students not only had the highest percentage selecting "parents" (84.2 percent) but were also the only group among Whites who selected "mother" more frequently than "father" or "parents." In this respect, Afrikaners once again resemble Blacks.

Turning to the second question in this sequence we asked the students to rank the three persons or groups whose evaluation of them *as a student* concerned them most. In 1974 Black students selected their parents, whereas Whites selected their teachers. In 1985 Blacks select their parents in almost the same way as they did before; White students in 1985 also selected their parents as most important. They gave "teacher" the nod in only 9.7 percent of the cases. This was in fact the lowest vote for teachers, who were selected by 18.3 percent of Indians (after parents), 17.4 percent of Blacks (after parents), and 16.9 percent of Coloureds (after parents).

Looking specifically at the White sample, we find that parents were selected by all four of the student categories. The status of the teacher had dropped in all cases, as well, and was selected in 10.2 percent of choices by both boys' and girls' schools, in 11.1 percent by Afrikaans students (down from 17.6 percent), and in only 8.5 percent of students in the fourth school. It is significant that whereas "teacher" had been selected in 41.3 percent of cases by the girls' school in 1974 (and parents had been selected by only 23.2 percent), a decade later only 10.2 percent made this same evaluation of teachers, and 75.0 percent selected "parents."

In 1974 there was a fairly clear leaning among the Blacks, and to a lesser extent among the Indians, toward members of the family and kin group. Among Whites, and to a lesser extent among

81

Coloureds, the emphasis was on the peer group and those persons outside the family, teacher or school principal, who are in positions of decision-making and authority. These findings suggested that Whites were less family oriented. In 1985 we saw a much greater emphasis on the opinion of parents, both in terms of ego as "person" and as "student." This means that friends (among White students), kinsmen (among Black and Indian students), and teachers (among Whites and especially White girls) had lost ground as the family reemerged as the core group for support and counsel.

Summary

It was significant that in two studies of White adolescents, one dealing with White males only and the other with high school seniors, we would have essentially the same percentages of users. While van der Burgh's data were somewhat prejudiced because he selected males only and most likely included persons who had already left school, his findings do serve as a baseline for us to compare the 1974 data.

Among Black students we find either nonuse or regular use. This is predictable because there was such a long tradition of cannabis and even institutionalization of its use with paraphernalia, idioms, and games. Persons who had a strong rural/traditional link or those who were strongly influenced by elders would then be more likely to smoke cannabis and to justify this on cultural-historical grounds.

Fairly early in this study the Afrikaans student emerged as the most conservative category—resembling in many ways Black students or English girls' school students. The reasons for this conservatism were complex but reached back into the Calvinist tradition and the contrast Afrikaners saw between themselves and their culture in comparison to the indigenous Blacks and their "primitive" practices. The interesting fact in 1985 was that Afrikaans and Black students vied with each other for the honor of being the most conservative. This was true also for the use of alcohol and for future plans or intended use of mind-altering substances.

An interesting pattern, applicable to all four of the sub-groups, emerged in discussing the peer group: the absence of a social clustering of users, and thus—one might suspect—the absence of a drug sub-culture. When we turned to alcohol use, however, we dealt with a legal drug so widely accepted that its presence was nearly universal and its use extremely common.

The last meaningful pattern which emerged from the foregoing discussion pertained to the "significant other." There was a change from 1974 in that most students in 1985 named their parents—or in the case of the Black and the Afrikaans students—the mother. When we moved beyond the home, we found a clear dichotomy in that Coloured and White high school seniors referred to their friends, while Black and Indian students referred to their kinsmen. This was to be expected in the two societies where lineages, extended family, kinship terminology, and patterned behavior was taught and recognized. Kinship bonds were real and were important on a daily basis.

5

CONTEXT OF CANNABIS AND ALCOHOL USE

Introduction

Human actions invariably involve human interactions. Behavior patterns are influenced as much by set as by setting. In looking at behavior involving the use of drugs, we must also look at the milieu, at parents and peers, at attitudes of approval or sanction, and at institutions which might influence the decision to experiment as much as the decision to use a substance. When we refer to "context," we mean the set—parents, peers, teachers, religious leaders, and others—as well as the setting—home, school, neighborhood, and so forth.

Parental attitudes and use of drugs

We were interested in knowing about the use of alcohol and cannabis and the attitude of the parents of students in our sample. Could we discern general tendencies which might influence either the acceptability or use of drugs? Alcohol was a legal drug and cannabis was not. How was this difference reflected in the actions and attitudes of parents? How were religious and traditional attitudes reflected?

The first question of the 1974 survey asked the students to indicate the normal pattern of alcohol use by their mothers and fathers. Among the respondents, 93.1 percent of the Indian students and 92.9 percent of the Black students indicated that their mothers never used alcohol. At the other end of the continuum, only 21.5 percent of the White sample stated that the mother never used alcohol. The Coloureds, with 56.3 percent, were in the middle of the two extremes. The same pattern showed up in response to the "regular use" variable: 13.6 percent of the

Whites and only 1.5 percent and 0.5 percent of the Indians and Blacks, respectively, indicated that their mothers used alcohol on a regular basis.

When we looked closely at the White sample, we found alcohol use was consistently higher among the English-speaking Whites than their Afrikaans speaking counterparts. The three English medium schools showed that in 15.5 percent, 21.4 percent, and 16.6 percent of the cases, the mother never used alcohol. The figure for the Afrikaans medium school was 38.6 percent. While 18.1 percent, 12.1 percent, and 15.2 percent of the students of English medium schools indicated regular use by their mothers, only 7.2 percent of the Afrikaans pupils selected this answer.

At the marginal English medium school, 4.3 percent of the students reported that their mothers used "considerable alcohol in social drinking"; 3.6 percent of the Afrikaans students came to this same conclusion. These figures rose to 10.7 percent and 6.9 percent, respectively, for the boys' and girls' schools in a wealthy, high-prestige neighborhood.

Alcohol use by the fathers presents the same pattern as that observed with the mothers. Table 14 presents this information for the four ethnic groups. Once again we find that Whites and Coloureds were the most common users of alcohol while the Black and Indian groups matched each other in most respects. A close look at the White sample (Table 15) indicates that the Afrikaans medium pupils felt that among their fathers were more teetotalers, fewer considerable social drinkers, and fewer persons who regularly used alcohol than figures for the other White group. While 43.4 percent of the Black students reported that their fathers abstained from alcohol in 1974, by 1985 the number had jumped to 69.0 percent reporting that their fathers drank no alcohol. At the same time, problem drinking among fathers rose for all ethnic groups. The English medium boys' and girls' schools had 15.6 percent and 15.7 percent, respectively, in which both parents were regular users of alcohol, "not in social situations only"; this figure for the Afrikaans school was only 8.5 percent.

Just as parental example influences choices and behaviors of youngsters who grow up in their parents' company or look up to them as role models, so, too, the attitude of parents will influence the behavior of children. Normally one can predict a lower incidence of alcohol use among young people who are raised in a

85

Table 14
PATTERN OF ALCOHOL USE BY FATHERS
OF HIGH SCHOOL SENIORS

Frequency	Black				Coloured				Indian				White			
	1974		1985		1974		1985		1974		1985		1974		1985	
	No.	%	No.	%	No.	%	No.	%	No.	%	No.	%	No.	%	No.	%
Not at all	84	43.4	80	69.0	21	25.9	67	38.1	127	40.7	131	39.2	54	11.3	38	9.3
Occasional social	66	34.1	15	12.9	19	23.5	54	30.7	105	33.7	114	34.1	246	51.5	206	50.4
Considerable social	11	5.6	4	3.4	15	18.5	15	8.5	21	6.7	17	5.1	54	11.3	61	14.9
Regular use	14	7.3	11	9.5	18	22.2	25	14.2	40	12.8	52	15.6	113	23.6	76	21.3
Problem drinking	9	3.9	6	5.2	5	6.2	15	8.6	11	3.5	20	6.0	13	2.2	17	4.2
NA	11	5.6			3	3.7			8	2.6			1	0.2		
Total	195	100.0	116	100.0	81	100.0	176	100.0	312	100.0	334	100.0	481	100.0	409	100.0
No response	33		10		8		4		25		7		17		3	

Table 15
PATTERN OF ALCOHOL USE BY FATHERS OF
WHITE HIGH SCHOOL SENIORS

Frequency	English Medium High School on City Outskirts				Afrikaans Medium Urban High School				English Medium Wealthy Neighborhood Boys School				English Medium Wealthy Neighborhood Girls School			
	1974		1985		1974		1985		1974		1985		1974		1985	
	No.	%	No.	%	No.	%	No.	%	No.	%	No.	%	No.	%	No.	%
Not at all	7	5.9	13	9.9	19	21.8	11	13.4	17	12.2	6	6.7	11	8.1	8	7.5
Occasional social	68	57.6	81	61.8	48	55.2	42	51.2	61	43.9	37	41.1	69	50.8	46	43.4
Considerable social	8	6.8	19	14.5	3	3.4	9	11.0	25	18.0	17	18.9	18	13.2	16	15.1
Regular use	32	27.1	15	11.5	13	14.9	14	17.1	33	23.7	27	30.0	35	25.7	31	29.2
Problem drinking	3	2.5	3	2.3	4	4.6	6	7.3	3	2.2	3	3.3	3	2.2	5	4.7
Total	118	100.0	131	100.0	87	100.0	82	100.0	139	100.0	90	100.0	136	100.0	106	100.0
No response	1		1		1				7				9		2	

home where alcohol either is not used or is used only on special social occasions. The same prediction can be made about the degree of acceptance or criticism with which student experimentation is met. These views are reflected in the attitudes of parents about students using alcohol.

A comparison of the students' impressions of their parents' views showed a considerable consistency over more than a decade. When the question was posed in 1974, the White students emerged as those who had the greatest freedom to use alcohol. Only 8.9 percent indicated their parents would be "intensely disapproving." In 1985 almost the same degree of approval was present, as 8.4 percent chose this category to represent their parents' attitudes. Among the Black students, 42.2 percent in 1974 and 43.2 percent in 1985 show about the same attitude as did the Coloureds of whom 44.9 percent in 1974 and 41.4 percent in 1985 thought their use of alcohol would be met with intense disapproval of their parents. For the Indians there was a much stronger religious and moral basis for not using alcohol. The Koran prohibits its use by Muslims; strict Hindus also accept prohibitions for its use. In this light it is only natural to find that 68.3 percent (in 1974) and 64.9 percent (in 1985) of the students expect their parents to disapprove intensely any use of alcohol. Much the same relationship between the four ethnic groups emerges when we look at those students who expect that their parents will be tolerant of alcohol use in social situations only. In 1974 as many as 54.9 percent of the Whites thought their parents would accept such use, and in 1985 this figure rose to 61.5 percent. The Black students also showed an increase from 11.4 percent to 13.6 percent over the intervening decade. There was a slight drop among Coloured students: 29.2 percent in 1974 and 27.2 percent in 1985. If Indians were the most disapproving it could be expected that they also would be less approving, even in social situations. The 9.5 percent in 1974 grew to 13.6 percent, the same figure as for the Black parents who were thought to approve of alcohol use a social context.

Turning to the use of cannabis, it should be recalled that what has become an accepted drug for White young people was viewed by the parental generation as something associated with "native" customs, degeneration, and degradation. Only the down and out smoked dagga. In time, as cannabis use was outlawed, a number of "confessions" appeared in the popular press, for example, by a "confirmed addict to bhang" (Harley-Mason 1938), by people who admit "I was a dagga smoker" (Bothma [ed.] 1951 and Godfrey 1955) or a "dagga slave" (Butch 1972). When we found in the 1974 survey that more than 90 percent of White students were sure that neither mother nor father had used cannabis, it really reflected the values of the parental generation and the aura associated with this illegal drug in contrast to their use of the legal drug, alcohol. In the 1985 survey there is a significant drop in the number of students who "know" that their parents have not experimented with cannabis. Only 79 percent could state this confidently.

When we turned our attention to the other ethnic categories included in this survey, the figures were lower only because in the eyes of the authorities such persons were members of socio-economic minority groups and were "guilty by association." Among Indians there were some traditions of use and even ritual context of use (see du Toit 1977[a]), yet their use of the drug in the view of their children was relatively low. Ninety-five percent of the mothers and 81 percent of the fathers were "known" not to have used cannabis. These figures once again held constant a decade later. The Coloureds were the group who had been the most marginal socially and culturally (Dickie-Clark 1966, 1972). One might have expected a greater degree of contact with Blacks and a greater emulation of their patterns of use. In 1974 we found that students thought 91 percent of their mothers but only 72.3 percent of their fathers had not used cannabis. A decade later 87 percent of the mothers and 69.7 percent of the fathers were known not to have used this drug. We should keep in mind that among Blacks, cannabis has been used for centuries. It was referred to as "the smoke of the ancestors"; it was associated with Chaka, the founder of the Zulu nation; it was used in ritual and ceremonial contexts by Zulu adults. An observer would then expect a greater use of cannabis among the parents of these Zulu youths. In the view of the students, their mothers and fathers were the most likely of the four ethnic groups to have used cannabis. This was true in 1974 and it was true in 1985, although the last figure for Whites and Blacks approach each other. It was of interest that 79.7 percent of the Black students and 78.6 percent of the White students "knew" that neither parent has used this drug, and that 6.5 percent of the Black and 6.8 percent of the White students were not sure of both parents. Although only 2.7 percent of the White students "knew" their parents had smoked cannabis, this figure rose to 8.1 percent for the Black students. The rest of the students are divided between knowing that one parent did and the other did not use this drug.

If we look specifically at the four White schools in the sample, it is interesting to note that the Afrikaans medium school in 1974 showed 100 percent of the pupils sure their mothers had never used cannabis. Students in the English medium White schools either suggested some previous use by mothers or not being sure. It is again the Afrikaans medium school students who indicate no cannabis use by any father with only one student unsure whether the father might have tried cannabis. Among the students in the other three schools, the figures for this question jumped to 7.8 percent and 8.6 percent for students in the two high-income, prestigious schools and 9.3 percent for the English medium school on the city outskirts. Students in these three schools were simply not convinced that their fathers had not used the drug in question. By 1985 we had little relative change. The Afrikaans medium school still had the highest percentage who knew their parents did not use cannabis; the boys' and girls' schools still had the lowest percentage of students who knew their parents did not use this drug. The position of "not sure" also remained the same: 6.7 percent and 6.5 percent of the boys' and girls' school, respectively, were not sure; but 8.4 percent of the city outskirts English school and only 4.9 percent of the Afrikaans school expressed this lack of conviction.

The next logical question which flows from this discussion is: What is the attitude of parents toward cannabis use by the high school seniors? The responses to this question appear in Table 16. In the 1974 findings the Coloured, Indian, and White parents appeared to be the most disapproving. In 1985 only the Indians retained this strong disapproval, and a higher percentage was seen as showing intense disapproval of cannabis use by their children. Among Black students we once again found ambivalence about a drug which had a long cultural history. Slightly over half the parents would strongly disapprove of its use; and almost one in six would be tolerant if their child, a high school senior, regularly smoked cannabis. These figures gain in importance if we keep in

Table 16
REACTION OF PARENTS TO CANNABIS USE
BY HIGH SCHOOL SENIORS

Reaction	Black				Coloured				Indian				White			
	1974		1985		1974		1985		1974		1985		1974		1985	
	No.	%	No.	%	No.	%	No.	%	No.	%	No.	%	No.	%	No.	%
Tolerant of regular use	6	2.8	17	17.5	0	0.0	0	0.0	3	0.9	4	1.2	2	0.4	2	0.5
Tolerant of trial only	5	2.3	7	7.2	0	0.0	1	0.6	3	0.9	5	1.5	18	3.7	16	3.9
Indifferent	33	15.5	12	12.4	2	2.2	2	1.1	8	2.4	6	1.8	2	0.4	4	1.0
Intense disapproval	138	64.8	52	53.6	82	92.1	144	81.8	204	88.8	299	89.3	422	86.6	338	82.8
Mixed different reactions	0	0.0			0	0.0			0	0.0			1	0.2		
Don't know	0	0.0			0	0.0			0	0.0			1	0.2		
NA	0	0.0			0	0.0			0	0.0			1	0.2		
Total	213	100.0	97	100.0	89	100.0	186	100.0	331	100.0	335	100.0	487	100.0	408	100.0
No response	15		29				4		6		6		11		4	

mind that the legal system in South Africa had not changed and that the Abuse of Dependence-Producing Substances and Rehabilitation Centres Act of 1971 and its 1973 amendment were enforced with the same stringency. In May 1971, Act 41 of 1971 became law. In the Schedule Part 1, a list of "prohibited dependence-producing drugs" appears which includes: cannabis, heroin, lysergide, mescaline, prepared opium, and others.

The first part of this Act deals with "dependence-producing drugs." It allows for a person who is found in possession of cannabis exceeding 115 grams in mass to be classified as dealing in this drug "unless the contrary is proven." It also refers to a person on whose land cannabis plants are found who then may be presumed to deal in this herb. In both cases a first conviction carried a penalty of "imprisonment for a period of not less than five years, but not exceeding fifteen years." In the case of a second or subsequent conviction the person may be imprisoned for a period of not less than ten years, but not exceeding twenty-five years. Conviction for use of cannabis carried a penalty of two to ten years imprisonment on first conviction and five to fifteen years on a second or subsequent conviction. Police are given the right to enter-and-search without warrant should they have "reasonable grounds" to suspect the presence or use of that drug or others. Enforcement is left to the discretion of the court and to the circumstances.

In contrast to the usual application of a law in which a person is considered innocent until proven guilty, the onus changes in this drug law. A person is now considered guilty until he can prove himself innocent. Article 10(3) states this explicitly: "If in any prosecution for an offense under this Act it is proved that any dependence-producing drug or plant from which such drug could be manufactured was found in the immediate vicinity of the accused, the accused shall be deemed to have been found in possession of such drug or plant, unless the contrary is proven." The implication of "immediate vicinity" was not clarified nor the evidence required to prove the contrary. A further complication in this case was that the state was not required to prove that it was in fact a dependence-producing drug or plant from which such could be prepared. Snyman (1974:29) in a detailed legal analysis of this law points out that "the practice in our courts in such cases is that it is sufficient to gain the opinion of a qualified person, such as a policeman, to accept that the substance was in fact dagga. . . ." Only in exceptional cases have the ipse dixit of such a "qualified" person been doubted and further proof required.

The first convictions under the new law occurred on December 9, 1971 when a magistrate in Pietermaritzburg sentenced seven Blacks who pleaded guilty to possessing cannabis. In each of the seven cases the magistrate found extenuating circumstances, and as provided by the law, did not impose the maximum sentences of five years. Punishment varied from twenty-one days to three months (suspended) for the adults and from four to six strokes for three youths aged nineteen and under. This shows that the magistrate could consider leniency.

The second part of the Act deals with matters of rehabilitation. Cannabis had been referred to separately in the first section, but it is not separately treated here. The presumption was that the cannabis user would be treated the same as the opium addict. (We intentionally selected these terms to imply aspects of habit formation, withdrawal symptoms, and tolerance, which are said not to be present in cannabis use.)

A new act, the Abuse of Dependence Procuring Substances and Rehabilitation Centres Amendment Act, became law in 1973. Its aim was to tighten up the original Drug Act. It prohibited the courts from imposing suspended sentences, postponing sentences, or discharging convicted persons with a caution or a reprimand. Persons over eighteen years of age who have assisted in the supply or traffic of the prohibited drugs thus were forced to go to jail.

The result of these two acts was a growing number of persons convicted for drug-related offenses. In the case of older people it meant removal from their families, losing their income and frequently their jobs, and the possibility of being relocated outside the urban environment where they had lived. For young persons imprisonment often meant being forced into association with hardened criminals. Numerous informants explained that after arrest for association with cannabis, they were actually forced to smoke it during imprisonment.

Through the combined and increased interest of police and law makers in the distribution and use of *Cannabis sativa* in southern Africa, a wedge had been driven between academic inquiry on one hand and official concern on the other. The grounds on which cannabis was included in the 1971 drug law

93

were insufficient, to say the least. In 1985, it was extremely difficult to get normal, spontaneous responses about patterns of distribution and use because of the very real fear of police infiltration, spying, and arrest. Rather than being able to conduct an inquiry about use and effect in the social setting of the community where users reside and work, studies were undertaken in the abnormal setting of institution or prison. The sole exception to such studies was the two-year research project, funded by the National Institute on Drug Abuse and carried out in the community by this writer between 1972 and 1974 (du Toit 1980[b]).

Discussing attitudes toward drugs, one of which was legal, the other illegal; one being introduced, the other traditional and simultaneously dealing with ethnic and cultural diversity called for sensitivity to the complexity of responses. Cannabis had certain religious and ritual uses in traditional Indian (particularly Hindu) society, but the use of alcohol was not sanctioned. This applied particularly to women. Although among the Blacks Xhosa women smoked, Zulus did not. Black women could use the mildly alcoholic but highly nutritious traditional brews, but they were not expected to use alcoholic beverages. Whites used alcohol in social and domestic contexts and smoked tobacco, with increasing numbers of women doing this, but to smoke cannabis was almost unthinkable. It was seen as a despicable practice associated with the "primitive" Black and one that was highly dangerous, resulting in detrimental conditions associated with altered consciousness and ultimately resulting in dependence.

Obviously, many young people did not share the views of their elders, and it was in this context that we asked students whether their parents used cannabis. In an analysis of the results, we found a large number of persons who indicated that they did not know whether their parents smoked cannabis. This was particularly true among the Black students. Adult males in these societies used to smoke a water pipe in the late afternoon much as their contemporaries who were White enjoyed a beer or some other drink. Since government intervention, cannabis smoking has been carried on covertly, and even the wife of a user is frequently oblivious to her husbands drug habit. For these reasons, and because of the history of drug use, we found that Blacks often did not know whether their parents smoked cannabis. There was not necessarily a relationship between parental use and student use. Coloured women showed up much more clearly as nonusers than their husbands, about whom there was some doubt. When we looked at the Indians and the Whites, we found the highest incidence of known parental cannabis use and a direct correlation between parental use of the drug and the use of cannabis by the student.

Social and religious organizations

Commenting on their findings in a study of a private northeastern U.S. seaboard college, Cheek and his associates (1973:335) stated that among users of cannabis "the majority were actively involved in extracurricular organized activities—social clubs and so forth." Du Toit and Suggs (1985) also found such normal involvement in social and cultural organizations by users of cannabis in a southern U.S. study. These findings were duplicated in the 1985 South African study. There was no clear distinction between user and nonuser as regards organizational or club activities.

Turning to participation in religious activities we again noticed a clear pattern influenced in part by ethnic group membership and in part by the fact that Indian religions allow many of the rituals to take place in the home. Our question which asked about attendance at religious worship services thus may not truly reflect religious activity. Nonetheless, we found a clear contrast between those who used cannabis and those who did not. Among the Black high school seniors in the 1974 study, 32.5 percent of those who used the drug never went to a religious service. Only 8.0 percent of those who did not use did not attend. This same picture emerges from the Coloured material, but the totals were small. The 27.3 percent who use and do not attend were therefore not as significant when contrasted with the 2.6 percent who did not use cannabis and did not attend. Again, the White students stood out as extremes. In this case they were the least religious or at least had the lowest attendance rate at religious services. Among the high school seniors, 26.8 percent of the cannabis users attended regularly, while 38.0 percent stated that they never attended. This compares with 39.1 percent and 23.8 percent, respectively, for the nonusers.

The clear pattern that emerged from the earlier findings, which was confirmed in the 1985 study, was that religious group participation and attendance at religious meetings (including worship services) was inversely correlated with cannabis use. As suggested earlier, this correlation may have been due to the practice of religiosity and attendance at religious services, but most likely it was due to the social context of non-users associated with religious group participation. It was not strange to find that in the Afrikaans medium school, students claimed simultaneously the highest incidence of nonuse of drugs (cannabis and alcohol) and the most regular participation in religious activities. The English boys' school presented the reverse picture of the lowest incidence of nonusers and the lowest religious participation. The Afrikaans school showed only 12.3 percent who were not religiously active and 95.1 percent who had not used cannabis. In contrast, the boys' school showed 44.4 percent who were not at all religiously active and only 63.3 percent who had not used cannabis.

Looking at this same material cross-culturally became more complicated. Nonusers were almost identical among Coloured, Indian, and Whites as a category; yet religious participation varied significantly because of the diversity of belief systems and forms of religious gatherings and worship. Blacks showed a pattern which most closely resembled that of the Afrikaans school students; Coloureds were much the same. The similarity can be explained partly by the denominational membership in Protestant and Catholic churches.

Friendship networks

To pursue the topic of the social network of drug users, we inquired about the best friends of our student subjects. Winick (1965) emphasized the smoking of cannabis as a social activity and the importance of sharing it with other young people. Bruce Johnson (1973) quite clearly described the American subculture of drug use. We asked the high school students how many of their best friends at home had smoked cannabis. It should be kept in mind that there was more than likely a larger percentage of students who smoked cannabis during the beginning or middle years of high school than during the final or senior years. Many of the drug users left school after standard eight (the tenth grade), going into technical colleges for practical job training or entering the labor market. Those who stayed on for the two senior years of high school were persons oriented toward furthering their education and tended to be more serious and less likely to use drugs. This sample could very well represent the smallest number of persons at the high school level who used cannabis.

Turning our attention to the high school seniors in 1974 (Table 17), we found that cannabis users among all four of the ethnic groups were more likely, by far, to have drug-using friends than was the case for non-using persons. For instance, slightly over 1 percent of nonusers had three close friends who smoked the drug. This figure rose to between 18 and 34 percent for users.

Within each ethnic group, we found that similar percentages of nonusing students claimed to have no drug using friends. In 1974, 84.6 percent of the Indian high school seniors claimed no close association with cannabis smokers. In 1985, a decade after the first survey, that figure has decreased slightly to 80.1 percent. It compared well with those for Black and White students, both categories having increased as more students apparently avoided close friendship with drug-using friends in the neighborhood.

It is important here, where we record responses of users and contrast them with those of nonusers, that strong correlations existed between individual use of drugs and the various attitudes and beliefs about those drugs. Seniors who used a given drug also were more likely to approve its use, downplay its risks, and report their own parents and friends as being at least somewhat more accepting of its use (Johnston et al. 1986:97, van der Burgh 1976:34).

Turning our attention to the other end of the scale is equally revealing. Users tended to have three best friends who used. Among Coloured students this figure had increased from 1974 and a decade later involved almost one in every four users. Among Indians the figure was about the same in the two surveys; one-in-five users had three best friends who used. Black and White students changed dramatically—but we should be reminded that the total figure for Black users was very low. Nevertheless, Blacks went from almost one-in-four users having three best friends who used to none, while Whites went from one-in-three to one-in-six. Looking at Table 17, it is interesting to note the comparison between users who had no drug-using friends when compared to

Table 17
HOW MANY OF YOUR BEST FRIENDS AT HOME HAVE SMOKED CANNABIS?

	Black				Coloured			
	1974		1985		1974		1985	
Number of Friends	User(%)	Non-user(%)	User(%)	Non-User(%)	User(%)	Non-user(%)	User(%)	Non-user(%)
None	10(25.6)	135(71.8)	4(50.0)	95(80.5)	2(18.2)	61(78.2)	18(26.5)	201(73.6)
One	6(15.4)	16(8.5)	1(12.5)	5(4.2)	2(18.2)	11(14.1)	15(22.1)	34(12.5)
Two	2(5.1)	9(4.8)	3(37.5)	3(2.5)	3(27.2)	2(2.6)	13(19.1)	7(2.5)
Three	9(23.1)	3(1.6)	0	4(3.4)	2(18.2)	1(1.3)	16(23.5)	7(2.5)
Don't Know	12(30.8)	25(13.3)	0	11(9.3)	2(18.2)	3(3.8)	6(8.8)	24(8.8)
Total	39(100.0)	188(100.0)	8(100.0)	118(99.9)	11(100.0)	78(100.0)	68(100.0)	273(99.9)

	Indian				White			
	1974		1985		1974		1985	
Number of Friends	User(%)	Non-user(%)	User(%)	Non-User(%)	User(%)	Non-user(%)	User(%)	Non-user(%)
None	26(39.4)	225(84.6)	9(26.5)	117(80.1)	17(23.9)	316(74.5)	23(30.6)	275(81.6)
One	13(19.7)	19(7.1)	6(17.6)	13(8.9)	13(18.3)	58(13.7)	15(20.0)	33(9.8)
Two	8(12.1)	6(2.3)	9(26.5)	4(2.7)	13(18.3)	22(5.2)	15(20.0)	10(3.0)
Three	15(22.7)	3(1.1)	7(20.6)	7(4.8)	24(33.9)	5(1.2)	12(16.0)	4(1.2)
Don't Know	4(6.1)	13(4.9)	3(8.8)	5(3.4)	4(5.6)	23(5.4)	10(13.3)	15(4.5)
Total	66(100.0)	266(100.0)	34(100.0)	146(99.9)	71(100.0)	424(100.0)	75(99.9)	337(100.1)

nonusers who have three drug-using friends. Without exception, users (who may use the drug secretly) are more likely to have friends who do not use than are nonusers likely to have best friends whom they know use cannabis.

An interesting similarity emerges in Tables 18 and 19 where the responses of Afrikaans-speaking Whites most closely approximated the responses of Black high school seniors. However, there is one glaring change. For some reason, exactly half of those who responded to the question (Table 19) would support the application of a known cannabis user for club membership, if all other criteria were met. This was the only student group in the 1985 study who would ignore to such a degree a person's use of this illegal drug. It might be a coincidence that 85.2 percent of this same student sample would persuade a close friend to stop smoking cannabis. Table 18 shows that this attitude was the highest among the four White student samples in both 1974 and 1985. These attitudes among Afrikaans speakers was most likely the result of a traditional, Calvinist-based philosophy, strong family orientation, and fear either of the stigma resulting from smoking a drug identified with the indigenous aboriginal population, or even more important, the possible stigma resulting from police confrontation. Among the Black students it was almost certainly related to fear of arrest and consciousness of having to get ahead in a country where the odds were against them. Education, good standing, and the absence of a police record were prerequisites for a Black person to "overcome" skin color, which engendered all kinds of legal and nonlegal differentiation and discrimination between people. These were also qualification essential for getting a decent job. The word "overcome" is used with reference to the White authority structure in South Africa and in full recognition of Black consciousness movements that were giving Blacks a new unity and a new pride. These movements were also active among students in both organized and spontaneous ways. While administering the survey questionnaire to the Black students in 1985, I was flanked by signs painted on the classroom wall, one proclaiming "Black Power !", the other "Free Mandela !". This last sign referred, of course, to Nelson Mandela, a prominent leader of the African National Congress who was serving a life sentence in jail. On February 11, 1990, after being incarcerated for 27 years, he was pardoned and freed.

Table 18
REACTION TO CANNABIS SMOKING BY CLOSE FRIEND

Reaction	English Medium High School on City Outskirts				Afrikaans Medium Urban High School				English Medium Wealthy Neighborhood Boys School				English Medium Wealthy Neighborhood Girls School			
	1974		1985		1974		1985		1974		1985		1974		1985	
	No.	%	No.	%	No.	%	No.	%	No.	%	No.	%	No.	%	No.	%
Disassociate	5	4.3	5	3.8	6	7.3	3	3.7	6	4.2	1	1.1	1	0.7	1	0.9
Decrease contact	6	5.2	10	7.6	1	1.2	2	2.5	7	4.9	3	3.3	7	4.8	4	3.7
Persuade to stop	76	66.1	99	75.6	72	87.8	69	85.2	93	64.6	55	61.1	107	73.8	89	83.2
Disregard use	28	24.3	17	13.0	3	3.7	7	8.6	38	26.4	31	34.4	30	20.7	13	12.1
Total	115	100.0	131	100.0	82	100.0	81	100.0	144	100.0	90	99.9	145	100.0	107	100.0
No response			1				1				1				1	

Table 19
WOULD YOU SUPPORT THE APPLICATION FOR CLUB MEMBERSHIP OF A PERSON KNOWN TO HAVE USED CANNABIS?

Response	English Medium High School on City Outskirts				Afrikaans Medium Urban High School				English Medium Wealthy Neighborhood Boys School				Girls School			
	1974		1985		1974		1985		1974		1985		1974		1985	
	No.	%	No.	%	No.	%	No.	%	No.	%	No.	%	No.	%	No.	%
Yes	64	53.8	51	39.2	22	25.3	41	50.0	62	43.1	32	36.0	98	67.6	33	30.6
No	27	22.7	38	29.2	45	51.7	25	30.5	48	33.3	33	42.7	27	18.6	36	33.3
Not sure	28	23.5	41	31.5	20	23.0	16	19.5	34	23.6	19	21.3	20	13.8	39	36.1
Total	119	100.0	130	99.9	87	100.0	82	100.0	114	100.0	84	99.9	145	100.0	108	100.0

These two groups, Blacks and Whites, clearly show what we may call "conformist attitudes." Drug use is a nonconformist activity when viewed against the general, ordered structure of society. However, when considered within the particular structure of the peer group or youth culture, it may be a conformist activity. This may explain some differences in the attitudes between White students at the English medium schools (especially the boys' school and the girls' school) who are most influenced by their peer group in contrast to the Black and Afrikaans students who are oriented toward and obviously influenced by their parents, their family, their religious community, and a wider social order.

Most cannabis users at school would be very secretive about the habit; but in the close social setting of a high school, news has a way of spreading. We were interested in the social implications of cannabis use. Would drug use cause social ostracism? To what extent would individuals accept or reject other individuals if they knew them to be drug takers? Or more practically, what would a person do if he discovered that a good friend of the same or opposite sex smoked cannabis? To elicit this information, a number of questions dealt with the social and personal implications of being a known cannabis smoker.

The first question sketched a situation in which a close personal friend began to use cannabis. The student was then asked to select a response from a number of alternatives. In the 1974 study a large majority of the Black (74.7 percent), Coloured (78.4 percent), Indian (79.1 percent), and White (71.6 percent) high school seniors stated that they would attempt to persuade their friends to stop. It is interesting that the Whites were lowest in this regard, thus suggesting either the belief that one is free to act as one pleases or a greater acceptance of the use of drugs. The next most common response to this question was that the student would disregard the friend's use of cannabis and it would not affect the friendship. Once again we found the highest percentage (20.4 percent) of Whites holding this opinion, while Coloureds (18.2 percent), Indians (14.3 percent) and Blacks (10.4 percent) found it less acceptable. At the other extreme were those high school students who stated that they would discontinue their friendship with a person found to be a cannabis smoker. Only one Coloured person indicated this choice, while 3.7 percent of the White students and 4.2 percent of the Indian students would act in this fashion. Black urban high school seniors were somewhat removed from the traditional Black culture and values and were committed to educational ideals espoused by the White culture; consequently 13.1 percent of them indicated that they would discontinue their friendship with a known cannabis smoker.

As can be seen in Table 18, the reactions of the Afrikaans students resemble those of the Black students. A very large majority would try to persuade a friend to stop smoking cannabis; very few would disregard the drug habit of a friend, and with the largest number of students of the four White schools, they would discontinue their friendship if they discovered that a friend smoked cannabis. However, when we examined the 1985 data, we found that the Afrikaans students had a more tolerant attitude. Although the vast majority (85.2 percent) would still try to persuade the person to stop using drugs, only 3.7 percent in 1985 as compared to 7.3 percent in 1974 would actually disassociate themselves from the user.

Peer-group importance

An idiom suggests that birds of a feather flock together. Stated differently, it is common to find a person selecting as friends people with whom he or she shares interests, activities, and values. This need not occur at the expense of kinship networks or family ties, but there frequently is a positive correlation between strains in or the absence of such networks and ties and the importance of the peer group. Vodra and Garbarino suggested that

> for older teenagers, the larger the percentage of kin included in the social network, the fewer behavior problems reported by mothers. Knowing the heterogeneity of the sample, it seems likely that the adolescents who were more disengaged from the kin network were those experiencing problems relating to home or school. It is possible that these teenagers turned to their peers in order to have their social needs met. And if, as is often the case, the peers to whom they turned were also disengaged from (or perhaps disillusioned with) their own families, the peer influence—or peer compensation—could have been negative in effect. (1988:217)

103

We turn now from friendship networks to the importance of peer group relationships. One way of measuring relationships within the peer group is to ask about willingness to date a person. Presumably dating occurs among persons with shared interests, background, and aims. People might be willing to date someone who has had an experience with an illegal drug, but they might not be willing to develop relationships with regular drug users. Looking at Table 20 we notice changes with reference to dating persons who had tried cannabis. Among Black, Coloured, and White seniors, the percentage of users who would date a user decreased; among the Coloureds and Whites, also, the nonusers who would date such a person had decreased between 1974 and 1985. During this decade, Indian users willing to date had increased, and Black and Indian nonusers were also more willing to date persons known to have used this drug. Except among the Black students, where figures were very low and may be meaningless, the "not sure" category had increased or remained the same over the decade among all the ethnic subcategories.

Dating a regular user was a different matter. Table 21 shows that students viewed this category in quite a different light. The first important fact that comes to light is the significant decrease among users and nonusers who would have been willing to date a user. As just one example, in 1985 84.0 percent of the White users would date a person who had tried cannabis; but only 26.7 percent would date a regular cannabis user. Indians retained about the same attitude as previously. Only the Coloured users in 1985 showed a greater percentage who were willing to date a user. The Indian students once again occupied a marginal position in that they were not sure of their views on dating a cannabis user. The combined result left the Indians with the smallest percentage among users and nonusers combined who would not date a drug user. This was strange given the family orientation and general conservatism we have noticed. By contrast the Coloureds were most likely to be affected negatively by the drug user as a possible date. Blacks are also quite negative in this regard. The White high school seniors evidenced both the smallest negative reaction to a date's drug use (among White users) and the greatest negative reaction among White nonusers.

104

Table 20
WOULD YOU DATE A PERSON WHO HAD TRIED CANNABIS?

	Black				Coloured			
	1974		1985		1974		1985	
Response	User(%)	Non-user(%)	User(%)	Non-User(%)	User(%)	Non-user(%)	User(%)	Non-user(%)
Yes	16(43.3)	26(14.1)	2(25.0)	21(17.8)	7(63.6)	25(32.5)	28(41.2)	44(16.1)
No	11(29.7)	96(52.2)	5(62.5)	69(58.5)	0(0.0)	20(26.0)	15(22.0)	115(42.1)
Not Sure	10(27.0)	62(33.7)	1(12.5)	28(23.7)	4(36.4)	32(41.5)	25(36.8)	114(41.8)
Total	37(100.0)	184(100.0)	8(100.0)	118(100.0)	11(100.0)	77(100.0)	68(100.0)	273(100.0)

	Indian				White			
	1974		1985		1974		1985	
Response	User(%)	Non-user(%)	User(%)	Non-User(%)	User(%)	Non-user(%)	User(%)	Non-user(%)
Yes	33(49.2)	54(20.2)	20(58.8)	39(26.7)	62(88.6)	180(43.2)	63(84.0)	124(36.8)
No	16(23.9)	116(43.5)	4(11.8)	42(28.7)	3(4.3)	99(23.7)	3(4.0)	88(26.1)
Not Sure	18(26.9)	97(36.3)	10(29.4)	65(44.5)	5(7.1)	138(33.1)	9(12.0)	125(37.1)
Total	67(100.0)	267(100.0)	34(100.0)	146(99.9)	70(100.0)	417(100.0)	75(100.0)	337(100.0)

Table 21
WOULD YOU DATE A REGULAR CANNABIS USER?

	Black				Coloured			
	1974		1985		1974		1985	
Response	User(%)	Non-user(%)	User(%)	Non-User(%)	User(%)	Non-user(%)	User(%)	Non-user(%)
Yes	14(36.8)	25(13.5)	1(12.5)	17(14.4)	1(9.1)	9(11.5)	13(19.1)	15(5.5)
No	9(23.7)	114(61.6)	5(62.5)	84(71.2)	6(54.5)	62(79.5)	46(67.6)	219(80.2)
Not Sure	15(39.5)	46(24.9)	2(25.0)	17(14.4)	4(36.4)	7(9.0)	9(13.2)	39(14.3)
Total	38(100.0)	185(100.0)	8(100.0)	118(100.0)	11(100.0)	78(100.0)	68(99.9)	273(100.0)

	Indian				White			
	1974		1985		1974		1985	
Response	User(%)	Non-user(%)	User(%)	Non-User(%)	User(%)	Non-user(%)	User(%)	Non-user(%)
Yes	15(22.7)	22(8.2)	8(23.5)	11(7.5)	36(50.7)	53(12.5)	20(26.7)	21(6.2)
No	41(62.1)	208(77.9)	14(41.2)	100(68.5)	22(31.0)	286(67.5)	30(40.0)	272(80.7)
Not Sure	10(15.2)	37(13.9)	12(35.3)	35(24.0)	13(18.3)	85(20.0)	25(33.3)	44(13.0)
Total	66(100.0)	267(100.0)	34(100.0)	146(100.0)	71(100.0)	424(100.0)	75(100.0)	337(99.9)

This same set of questions was asked by Grupp, McCain, and Schmitt (1971) in their study of students in a U.S. Midwest college. They found that 95 percent of the users and 64 percent of the nonusers would be willing to date a person who was known to have experimented with cannabis. Willingness to date a regular user of this drug declined to 61 percent of the users and only 15 percent of the nonusers. These figures would approximate most closely the 1974 figures for Whites. By 1985 even this category of respondents had become more cautious or conservative about interpersonal relations.

Summary

This chapter has discussed the use of cannabis and alcohol in its social context, the former context translating into an illegal one based on the Abuse of Dependence-Producing Substances and Rehabilitation Centres Act (1971). Social context involved parents, the domestic arrangement, social and religious organizations, as well as friendship networks—both those operating in the residential neighborhood and those pertaining to the school setting.

On the whole, we found nonuse of cannabis by mothers in all four ethnic samples but especially Black and Indian. Alcohol use was also consistently lower among mothers, least so among Whites. Among the Whites, however, we found the Afrikaners emerging as the overall most conservative group. This pertained not only to expected use by parents but also to parental attitudes concerning experimentation or drug use by the students.

Although high school seniors were quite clear in their selection of friends and dates as to whether such persons used drugs and would in most cases try to convince a using friend to refrain from such activity, they did not distinguish drug use in club membership. Even the most conservative Afrikaans students in more than half the cases, would have supported the membership of a person who was known to use drugs. There seemed to be quite a clear differentiation between being acquainted with or being a friend of somebody who had used an illegal substance in contrast to dating such a person. Even clearer was the distinction between dating a person who had experimented versus one who used mind-altering substances.

Finally, there was a clear coincidence between religiosity and nonuse. What we see here is a composite of associational factors in which peer group, social group networks, religiosity, and parental influence all interact. As Bruce Johnson has pointed out "The strong relationship between religiosity and cannabis use exists mainly because less religious persons become involved in peer groups where cannabis is used and hence use the drug themselves" (1973:61). Once again we found the Black high school seniors clearly contrastive with the other ethnic groups. We also saw the Afrikaans students differ from the other White schools—especially the boys' school—and the great similarity between the conservative Blacks and the Afrikaans students.

6

STUDENT ATTITUDES ON CANNABIS
AND ALCOHOL USE

Introduction

A major part of the survey questionnaire dealt with the attitudes of high school seniors toward the use, effects, legal position, and related matters pertaining to students who used either the illegal drug, cannabis, or the legal drug, alcohol. Of some interest were the differing views held by users versus nonusers of these drugs. However, since the user category was frequently quite small and contrasting views might thus lose significance, it was interesting to look at the views of different ethnic categories of high school seniors about the use of drugs.

> When considering the attitudes of young people toward drug use it is important to look not just at the attitude of a number of individuals but at the social context of the people concerned, the movement or value system which is their primary reference group and the way in which drugs are used in that group. (Hartnoll and Mitcheson 1973:15)

We have established that the students had friendship relationships, dating, and peer interaction, and that they had both school friends and home friends. With this social context confirmed and the cultural background and ethnicity located in the South African social mosaic, we can explore attitudes held by high school seniors.

Reasons for drug use

The questionnaire turned at this stage to the reasons why pupils had or had not used cannabis. The questions permitted a fairly wide range of choices, and the pupils were verbally instructed that they could make more than one selection. The first question asked: "If you have never tried dagga, what are your reasons for not trying it?"

In the 1974 study, the most common reason given was a lack of interest in the drug, and this reason was fairly evenly distributed among the four ethnic samples. As the second most common reason, the Black students claimed lack of access to the drug and the physical and mental risks to which cannabis users exposed themselves. This reason, along with parental influence, was also listed by White students. Parental influence was also important among the Indian and Coloured seniors, the latter also mentioning moral and religious reasons for avoiding the use of cannabis.

Not all the pupils elected to give more than one reason, but among those who did, physical and mental risks emerged as a critical factor. Risk was mentioned by 38.1 percent of the Blacks, 63.6 percent of the Coloureds, 64.0 percent of the Indians, and only 33.0 percent of the Whites. In those cases where pupils gave three reasons for not trying cannabis, this fear of detrimental physical and mental effects was mentioned as the overwhelming reason.

The results of the 1985 survey confirmed many of our earlier findings. All the students, with the exception of Blacks, indicated a lack of interest as justification for nonexperimentation and nonuse. This reason was the most common among the Coloureds. Almost as frequently mentioned among Indian and White students were the health risks taken by a drug user. This reason was the second most frequently mentioned by the Coloured students. It will be remembered that among Indian students the peer group was a significant reference group. Here again we find that friends' influence was an important reason why Indian students did not experiment with drugs. Secondary reasons listed by Whites were fear of physical dependence and fear of addiction.

It should be stated at this juncture that at the time of these studies (1974 and 1985) there were no formal drug education programs in the schools. Individual teachers no doubt spoke about the subject, but a student's knowledge would come from church, formal national programs in the press, on radio and on television, or informal street wisdom.

A second question, aimed at those students who had experimented with or were using drugs, asked students to "indicate the one main reason for doing so." We were dealing specifically with the use of cannabis. Curiosity, as can be seen in Table 22, was the most common reason given by Blacks, Coloureds, and Indians. This finding agreed with that of Gomberoff and his colleagues (1972:31) who found that for adolescents in Chile "curiosity is one of the most important motivations to smoke marihuana." Curiosity was not the primary reason among the White high school seniors in 1974, though it became so a decade later.

One alternative on the list presented to the students in the questionnaire was "expression of resistance to the Establishment." In 1974 no Coloured or Indian student, and only one Black student, gave this as the reason for smoking cannabis. Among the Whites, 12.5 percent explained their drug use as a reactionary decision against the Establishment, including authority figures and disciplinary conditions at school and at home. Interestingly, in 1985 this reason completely disappeared as not a single student selected it. This should be seen in the context in which parents were listed as the most important persons in the lives of students; persons whose evaluation of the "student" and the "person" are most highly valued.

Among students at the four White high schools "resistance" was the primary reason given in 1974 for cannabis use by girls at the highly prestigious girls' school. They selected this reason almost four times as frequently as any other. Among the boys at the highly prestigious boys' school, "curiosity" slightly outranked "resistance" as was the case among students in the English medium school on the city outskirts. It was strange that among the more conservative students at the Afrikaans medium school, one mentioned "curiosity," one explained that the drug had been used for "kicks—to feel good," but ten students indicated that they had used cannabis as an expression of "resistance." This finding was somewhat of an anomaly because the overall picture which emerged from the 1974 study was that the Afrikaans student was much more accepting of the status quo, of authority figures, of the

111

Table 22
PRIMARY REASON GIVEN BY HIGH SCHOOL SENIORS
FOR TRYING CANNABIS

Reason	Black 1974 No.	%	Black 1985 No.	%	Coloured 1974 No.	%	Coloured 1985 No.	%	Indian 1974 No.	%	Indian 1985 No.	%	White 1974 No.	%	White 1985 No.	%
Never used	143	76.1	118	93.7	69	86.1	146	81.1	224	77.5	274	80.4	332	72.8	337	81.8
Curiosity	22	11.7	3	2.4	6	7.5	20	11.1	35	12.1	42	12.3	32	7.9	45	10.9
Kicks—to feel good	7	3.7	1	0.8	3	3.8	3	1.7	15	5.2	10	2.9	19	4.2	16	3.9
Escape problems	5	2.7	1	0.8	0	0.0	1	0.6	6	2.1	4	1.2	3	0.7	3	0.7
Social pressures	1	0.5	1	0.8	1	1.3	2	1.1	4	1.4	5	1.5	5	1.1	5	1.2
Self-understanding	4	2.1	1	0.8	1	1.3	2	1.1	2	0.7	0	0.0	1	0.2	1	0.2
Resistance	1	0.5	0	0.0	0	0.0	0	0.0	0	0.0	0	0.0	57	12.5	0	0.0
Relaxation	0	0.0	0	0.0	0	0.0	1	0.6	2	0.7	3	0.9	0	0.0	0	0.0
Boredom	1	0.5	0	0.0	0	0.0	5	2.8	0	0.0	1	0.3	0	0.0	2	0.5
Intensify perception	1	0.5	0	0.0	0	0.0	0	0.0	0	0.0	0	0.0	0	0.0	1	0.2
Other	3	1.6	1	0.8	0	0.0	0	0.0	1	0.3	2	0.6	3	0.7	2	0.5
Total	188	99.9	126	100.0	80	100.0	180	100.1	289	100.0	341	100.1	452	100.1	412	99.9
No response	40				9				48				42			

112

role of parents and similar issues. Perhaps those few who do not fit intended to act it out radically in such ways as using drugs.

We can state, in general, that among White high school seniors in 1974, cannabis had lost some of its stigma and had become a symbol of resistance. As seniors two decades earlier had used alcohol to express independence and to affirm their new status or as seniors two decades before them used cigarettes, the current high schoolers in 1974 used cannabis. They might have been curious about it, but it also represented reaction to authority. In 1985 the social and political climate in the country had changed. Cannabis, in spite of its illegality, was no longer a substance surrounded by an aura of the unknown. Resistance against parental and other authority figures had waned. Fewer students used cannabis and those who did were motivated mainly by curiosity. In 1985 curiosity was listed as the reason for using cannabis by 52.2 percent of the English school, 50.0 percent of the Afrikaans school, 60.6 percent of the boys' school, and 73.3 percent of the girls' school senior students. Trailing as a distant second reason was "kicks—an enjoyable experience, to feel good." The only other reason to emerge as vaguely significant was the use of the drug to cope with social pressure, indicated as peer pressure, and the need to be "in" with friends. This was also an important evaluation for the Indian students.

Believed characteristics of drug users

As part of the attitude survey, high school seniors were asked to characterize cannabis users. They were presented with a list of characteristics which allowed them to make positive, neutral, or negative evaluations. It must be emphasized that a dagga smoker in South African folk traditions had a very negative image. Such a person was frequently described as dull, morally degenerate, not physically active, and the kind of person who flunked out of school during his middle teens.

The responses of students in 1974 (Table 23) indicated that the variable which states "not much different from people who do not use it" was selected most frequently. The sole exception here were the Coloureds, a small majority of whom selected the variable which reads "in need of psychiatric help." This was also the second most frequent choice among the Indian students. The Black

Table 23
CHARACTERISTICS OF THE AVERAGE CANNABIS
USER AS VIEWED BY HIGH SCHOOL SENIORS

Characteristic	Black				Coloured				Indian				White			
	1974		1985		1974		1985		1974		1985		1974		1985	
	No.	%	No.	%	No.	%	No.	%	No.	%	No.	%	No.	%	No.	%
Same as non-users	69	32.1	20	15.9	23	25.8	70	40.9	103	31.3	81	24.5	214	44.5	157	39.2
Sensitive-intelligent	35	16.3	23	18.3	2	2.2	4	2.3	28	8.5	19	5.7	12	2.5	6	1.5
Poor students	29	13.5	24	19.0	14	15.7	15	8.8	47	14.3	49	14.8	74	15.4	43	10.7
Lower class	35	16.3	24	19.0	8	9.0	15	8.8	44	13.4	49	14.8	33	6.9	43	10.7
Morally degenerate	16	7.4	10	8.0	13	14.6	18	10.5	35	10.6	33	10.0	53	11.0	47	11.7
Psych. cases	14	6.5	21	16.6	24	27.0	36	21.1	52	15.8	75	22.7	48	10.0	60	15.0
Other	13	6.0	4	3.2	4	4.5	13	7.6	17	5.2	25	7.5	45	9.4	45	11.2
Don't know	4	1.9			1	1.1			3	0.9			2	0.2		
Total	215	100.0	126	100.0	89	99.9	171	100.0	329	100.0	331	100.0	481	99.9	401	100.0
No response	13				9		9		8		10		17		11	

students, in equal numbers, decided that cannabis users were "more sensitive and intelligent than the average" and that they were "mostly from a lower-class background." A decade later fewer high school seniors from the same schools viewed drug users as the same as nonusers (except for the Coloured students). The Indian and White students suggested that persons who smoke cannabis were "in need of psychiatric help," that they tended to derive "mostly from a lower-class background," and that they were "mainly students who do poorly in school." The White students also indicated as a third characteristic what they perceived as a moral degeneration in drug users. The Coloured students, in spite of the fact that more now saw cannabis smokers as "not much different from people who do not use it," selected the same social and psychological characteristics to describe drug users as did Indians and Whites. Black students, deriving from ghetto living conditions and the heterogeneity of social classes, traditionalists, and educated people, seemed much less sure of the characterization. Fewer saw them as the same as nonusers and almost equal percentages saw persons who smoke dagga as poor students and conversely, as "more sensitive and intelligent than the average." It should be emphasized that this latter category was selected in 1974 by more Black students (16.3 percent) than the other three ethnic groups combined.

Looking more closely at the White students, the primary characteristic ascribed to drug users by the English medium co-educational school was that they were poor students (16.0 percent); the boys' school describes them as "lower class" (13.6 percent). The girls' school students saw the drug user as morally degenerate (17.6 percent) and in need of psychiatric aid (13.9 percent) while the Afrikaans students saw psychiatric help (25.0 percent) as indicated for such persons who usually derive from lower-class backgrounds (17.5 percent).

Turning from the moral-intellectual characteristics, pupils were asked whether cannabis users were physically active or passive types. Black, Coloured, and Indian high school seniors all agreed with very slight variations that there was not much difference between users and nonusers. The 1974 White students differed quite markedly from the other ethnic groups. While 49.3 percent said that cannabis users were not much different from other people, 41.8 percent saw the cannabis smoker as a "physically inactive, passive type," and only 9 percent thought they were "physically active, sporting types." The other ethnic groups among our high school seniors had chosen each of these three alternatives with about equal frequency. In 1985 the Whites (50.5 percent) and Coloureds (46.1 percent) thought that users and nonusers were quite equal in terms of physical activity. However, most students from the total sample thought that "people who use dagga [were] on the average physically inactive, passive types." This was the second choice of Coloured (41.7 percent) and White (43.7 percent) students, and the first choice of Indian (41.3 percent) students. Black students were very evenly split. A small majority (35.7 percent) thought that cannabis users were less active than other students, but 29.4 percent saw them as the same and 29.4 percent saw them as more active than nonusers (5.6 percent did not respond to this question). The last figure was very interesting, especially when it was contrasted with a mere 4.8 percent of the White students who saw cannabis smokers as "physically active sporting types." This view among Black students could have derived from the fact that professional soccer players and musicians, both of whom are greatly admired because they have essentially straddled the racial barrier, are said to smoke cannabis quite openly and regularly.

When we look at the four White schools, the Afrikaans medium high school once again showed the clearest contrast in the 1974 responses (Table 24). In 1985, however, students at the boys' (64.0 percent) and girls' (57.4 percent) schools in the prestigious White suburb reaffirmed their view that drug users and nonusers were not much different in levels of activity. Students at the coeducational school (51.9 percent) indicated that they saw cannabis smokers as being physically less active. Neither category of students thought that drug users were "physically active, sporting types." This left us with the Black students as the sole exceptions who viewed cannabis smokers in this light.

Believed risks in drug use

To expand the attitudinal scope of the survey, a number of questions asked students to what risks they thought a cannabis user was exposed. Related to this question was one which explored the social and interpersonal implications of drug use. In

Table 24
PERCEPTION OF CANNABIS SMOKERS BY
WHITE HIGH SCHOOL SENIORS

Characteristic	English Medium High School on City Outskirts				Afrikaans Medium Urban High School				English Medium Wealthy Neighborhood Boys School				English Medium Wealthy Neighborhood Girls School			
	1974		1985		1974		1985		1974		1985		1974		1985	
	No.	%	No.	%	No.	%	No.	%	No.	%	No.	%	No.	%	No.	%
Physically active	13	12.5	8	6.2	5	6.7	3	3.7	21	14.8	5	5.6	3	2.1	4	3.7
Physically inactive	30	28.2	67	51.9	51	68.0	44	53.7	46	32.4	27	30.3	68	46.9	42	38.9
No difference	62	59.4	54	41.9	19	25.3	35	42.7	75	52.8	57	64.0	74	51.0	62	57.4
Total	105	100.0	129	100.0	75	100.0	82	100.1	142	100.0	89	99.9	145	100.0	108	100.0
No response	14		3		13				4		1					

the first of these questions, a number of possible risks were listed; the students were asked to "indicate which of the following you feel is a risk taken by anyone who uses dagga." More than one choice was permitted, but the majority of the respondents selected only one item (Table 25). In the 1974 study all four of the ethnic groups recognized damage to health as the most immediate risk; the Coloured (75.3 percent) and Indian (71.9 percent) high school seniors were more concerned about this danger than were their Black and White counterparts. A decade later, Blacks (71.4 percent) were most concerned about health, and Indians saw health risks (38.9 percent) and possible addiction (37.2 percent) as the greatest threats to a cannabis user. Coloured students were also fearful of addiction (44.4 percent) and a number of other potential harmful effects. The most adverse response pattern was found among the Whites: these students in almost equal numbers recognized damage to health (26.5 percent); escalation to the use of hard drugs (24.8 percent); and addiction (23.1 percent) as risks. These figures derived from an English medium coeducational school where 48.1 percent saw a danger to health, and two English medium schools, one for boys and one for girls. In both of the latter, escalation to hard drugs was seen as the greatest risk courted by a cannabis user.

Related to risk in a physical sense are the social implications of drug use. How does the known use of an illegal substance affect the acceptance of such people by their peers? Would others date such a person, or would they support such a person in areas away from the use of the drug? Students were asked whether they would date a person known to have experimented and also whether they would date a regular cannabis user. We found an interesting response pattern among Whites. In the 1985 survey (figures for 1974 appear in parentheses), we found that 74.2 percent (52.9 percent) of the seniors at the English medium coeducational school indicate that they would not date a person known to be a user. A similar increase was found at the girls' school with 77.8 percent (57.2 percent), while the Afrikaans medium school remained the most conservative with 80.5 percent (77.0 percent) of seniors not willing to date a drug user. Only the students at the boys' school showed a willingness to date girls who smoked cannabis as only 60.0 percent indicated they would not; equally significant is the fact that this figure is down from 66.2

118

Table 25

RISKS TAKEN BY PERSONS SMOKING CANNABIS AS
SEEN BY HIGH SCHOOL SENIORS

Risk	Black 1974 No.	%	Black 1985 No.	%	Coloured 1974 No.	%	Coloured 1985 No.	%	Indian 1974 No.	%	Indian 1985 No.	%	White 1974 No.	%	White 1985 No.	%
Damage to health	156	69.0	90	74.4	67	75.3	44	27.2	240	71.9	132	42.6	333	67.4	109	29.7
Physical dependence	8	3.5	5	4.1	1	4.5	10	6.2	14	4.2	17	5.5	28	5.7	31	8.4
Psychological dependence	15	6.6			3	3.4			24	7.2			45	9.1		
Legal sanctions	20	8.8	9	7.4	3	3.4	7	4.3	7	2.1	5	1.6	27	5.5	19	5.2
Addiction	10	4.4	1	0.8	9	10.1	80	49.4	41	12.3	126	40.7	31	6.3	95	25.9
Escalation	9	4.0	2	1.7	3	3.4	18	11.1	4	1.2	24	7.7	26	5.3	102	27.8
Don't know	2	0.9														
No risk	6	2.7	14	11.6	0	0.0	2	1.2	4	1.2	6	1.9			6	1.6
Other			0	0.0			1	0.6			0	0.0	4	0.8	5	1.3
Total	226	99.9	121	100.0	86	100.1	162	100.0	334	100.1	310	100.0	494	100.1	367	99.9
No response	2		5				18		3		31		4		45	

percent in 1974. Exactly the same pattern was evident in the "not sure" category: the coeducational school showed 16.7 percent (29.4 percent) and the girls' school 11.1 percent (21.4 percent) who had reservations about dating a cannabis user. The Afrikaans students have few reservations, as only 8.5 percent (9.2 percent) were hesitant. The boys' school shows a significant increase in this category as 31.1 percent (16.6 percent) of the seniors were not sure about dating a girl who smoked cannabis.

A further question in the area of social relations, touches on the degree to which a person's experimentation with or use of an illegal drug might influence social acceptance. Would such a person face ostracism? We do know that persons who use drugs tend to associate with other such persons, but is this by choice or social pressure?

The last question in our series which tried to gauge the social implications of cannabis smoking asked whether the pupil would support the application to join a social club of another pupil who was known to have tried cannabis. The result in 1974 showed that 49.7 percent of the White students and 53.4 percent of the Coloured students would accept cannabis users into their organization. They were clearly the least concerned about the drug use of a friend. Ten years later, however, students had become more conservative. Then only 40.2 percent of the Coloured and 33.3 percent of the Whites would indiscriminately admit students to their social club. Indian students in 1974 were almost bimodal as 38.8 percent versus 36.1 percent indicated they would versus would not admit a known drug user to a social club. In 1985, 35.3 percent indicated they would admit a user, 31.8 percent said they would not, and 32.9 percent were not sure what decision they would make if confronted with a choice. Black students were clearly not supportive of cannabis smokers. In 1974 only 27.9 percent said they would support such an application while 50.9 percent would oppose it. In 1985 only 23.0 percent would support it in contrast to 62.7 percent who would not. This last figure was twice as high as the Coloured and Indian percentages and significantly higher than the Whites.

Turning to a detailed analysis of White students, Table 26 shows relatively little change in the relative evaluations of the Afrikaans students and the seniors at the boys' school. However, significantly lower percentages of students in the coeducational school and the girls' school would support such an application in 1985 than had been the case ten years before. In fact, both categories had decreased by almost one-half. The student group which was least influenced by drug use of club members in 1985 were the seniors at the English boys' school.

In a review of trends of drug use among high school students in the United States, Johnston and his associates found that

> from 1975 through 1978 there had been a decline in the harmfulness perceived to be associated with all levels of marijuana use; but in 1979, for the first time, there was an increase in these proportions—an increase which preceded any appreciable downturn in use and which has continued fairly steadily since then. By far the most impressive increase has occurred for *regular marijuana use*, where there has been a full 32% jump in just five years in the proportion perceiving it as involving great risk—i.e., from 35% in 1978 to 67% in 1984. This is a dramatic change, which continued vigorously in 1984 with a 4% increment, and it has occurred during a period in which a substantial amount of scientific and media attention has been devoted to the potential dangers of heavy marijuana use. While there have been some upward shifts in concerns about the harmfulness of occasional, and even experimental, use, they have been nowhere nearly as large, though both did continue in 1984. (Johnston et al. 1985:100)

This negative evaluation translated into strong disapproval of use at any level. Since 1977 there had been disapproval of experimentation, occasional use and regular use; this disapproval rate continued to rise. In a later survey, these same researchers reported that regular cannabis use was "judged to involve great risk by 70% of the sample" (Johnston et al. 1986:111).

In the case of alcohol use we found a large number of users and a tendency to justify use based on the student's own behavior. While 73 percent disapproved of one or two drinks on a daily basis, binge drinking on weekends was acceptable to a much greater percentage. The reason was that this latter pattern

Table 26

WOULD YOU SUPPORT THE APPLICATION FOR CLUB MEMBERSHIP
OF A PERSON YOU KNEW HAD USED "DAGGA"?

Response	English Medium High School on City Outskirts				Afrikaans Medium Urban High School				English Medium Wealthy Neighborhood Boys School				English Medium Wealthy Neighborhood Girls School			
	1974		1985		1974		1985		1974		1985		1974		1985	
	No.	%	No.	%	No.	%	No.	%	No.	%	No.	%	No.	%	No.	%
Yes	64	53.8	38	29.2	22	25.3	25	30.5	62	43.1	38	42.7	98	67.6	36	33.3
No	27	22.7	51	39.2	45	51.7	41	50.0	48	33.3	32	36.0	27	18.6	33	30.6
Not sure	28	23.5	41	31.5	20	23.0	16	19.5	34	23.6	19	21.3	20	13.8	39	36.1
Total	119	100.0	130	99.9	87	100.0	82	100.1	114	100.0	89	100.0	145	100.0	108	100.0

agreed with their own pattern of use and thus was justified based on their own behavior.

Control of drug use

An area of concern to many people pertains to appropriate legal control of cannabis use and also legal action against persons found guilty of drug use. In the first of the questions pertaining to legality, students were asked what degree of legal control they felt was appropriate for cannabis. The Black students differed quite clearly from the other three groups (Table 27). As was the case in 1974, so ten years later the Black students were still the group who found greatest justification for having no legal restrictions on the use of this drug. All three of the other groups confirmed the position taken in 1974 that cannabis should not be legal and that penalties should stay as they were. Not only did these students confirm their primary selection, they also confirmed the relative response pattern created by seniors from their same schools a decade previously.

Moving from appropriate legal control and possible decriminalization of cannabis, we inquired what these students thought would be appropriate legal action if a person were found guilty of cannabis use. Table 28 suggests that being sent to jail was a form of punishment which had become less popular among all the groups and while it still was seen as appropriate by a large number of Blacks this may have been due to socialization and experience—few of them would have a close relative who had not been jailed for some reason. The alternative to incarceration was that the person be warned and then released. This was seen by Black students as the most appropriate legal action, but their counterparts in the other student groups did not give this alternative high rating.

Indian and White students, and to a slightly lesser extent the Coloureds, selected rehabilitation as the appropriate action. The item in the questionnaire read: "Made to report regularly to a rehabilitation center." Their belief apparently was that this would change the habit of the user, but Black students did not in 1974, nor did they ten years later, give it much preference.

American students, when surveyed about the legal status of cannabis in 1985, appeared only slightly more liberal than the

123

Table 27

APPROPRIATE LEGAL CONTROL FOR CANNABIS USE
AS SEEN BY HIGH SCHOOL SENIORS

Legal Control	Black				Coloured				Indian				White			
	1974		1985		1974		1985		1974		1985		1974		1985	
	No.	%	No.	%	No.	%	No.	%	No.	%	No.	%	No.	%	No.	%
No legal restrictions	51	23.1	35	28.0	11	12.4	15	8.4	33	10.0	32	9.4	34	7.0	36	8.7
Legal if over age 21	30	13.6	18	14.4	2	2.2	11	6.2	36	10.9	22	6.5	37	7.6	30	7.3
Legal for experiments and research	65	29.4	31	24.8	36	40.4	55	30.9	105	31.8	84	24.7	139	28.5	70	17.0
Reduced penalties	31	14.0	12	9.6	3	3.4	19	10.7	34	10.3	33	9.7	83	17.0	41	10.0
Same penalties	28	12.7	21	16.8	37	41.6	78	43.8	120	35.9	169	49.7	180	37.0	234	56.8
OK for non-whites	8	3.6	3	2.4	0	0.0	0	0.0	3	0.9	0	0.0	5	1.0	1	0.2
OK for Africans	8	3.6	5	4.0	0	0.0	0	0.0	1	0.3	0	0.0	9	1.8	0	0.0
Total	221	100.0	125	100.0	89	100.0	178	100.0	332	100.1	340	100.0	487	99.9	412	100.0
No response	7		1				2		6		1		11		1	

124

Table 28

APPROPRIATE PUNISHMENT FOR A PERSON FOUND
GUILTY OF CANNABIS USE

Punishment	Black				Coloured				Indian				White			
	1974		1985		1974		1985		1974		1985		1974		1985	
	No.	%	No.	%	No.	%	No.	%	No.	%	No.	%	No.	%	No.	%
Sent to jail	99	44.0	40	32.5	11	12.6	13	7.2	55	16.4	51	15.0	56	11.5	37	9.0
Physical punishment	24	10.7	12	9.8	3	3.4	11	6.1	21	6.3	8	2.4	31	6.3	3	0.7
Fined	21	9.3	7	5.7	10	11.5	20	11.1	3	13.1	25	7.4	75	15.3	43	10.5
Rehabilitated	11	4.9	7	5.7	51	58.7	105	58.3	131	39.1	216	63.7	213	43.6	258	62.8
Warned and released	53	23.5	43	35.0	9	10.3	20	11.1	68	20.3	25	7.4	60	12.3	47	11.4
Other	17	7.6	14	11.4	3	3.4	11	6.1	16	4.8	14	4.1	54	11.0	23	5.6
Total	225	100.0	123	100.0	87	100.0	180	100.0	294	100.0	339	100.0	489	100.0	411	100.0
No response	3		3		2				2		2		9		1	

majority of South African high school seniors. Johnston and his associates found that "less than one-fifth of all seniors believe[d] marijuana use should be entirely legal (17%). About one out of four (26%) [felt] it should be treated as a minor violation—like a parking ticket—but not as a crime. Another 17% indicate[d] no opinion, leaving about two-fifths (41%) who [felt] it still should be treated as a crime" (1986:123). These figures were closest to the position of the Coloured students, where about 15 percent would place no legal restrictions (especially on adults), 11 percent saw it as a minor violation which should imply reduced penalties, and 44 percent would maintain the status quo with the same penalties. The other 31 percent in our survey would see cannabis used in experimental and research situations. The other ethnic categories in our research were more conservative.

Summary

To use or not to use, that was the question. The majority who decided not to use based their decision on lack of interest or fear of risk factors. The increase in a consciousness of the latter suggested a better informed and more sophisticated group of twelfth graders than existed a decade previously. Curiosity remained a primary reason for experimenting.

In 1974, there were clear strains in social relations. Young people were looking outside the family for significant others, peer group members were of great importance, friendship ties in many cases were given priority over family ties, and cannabis was smoked as an expression of resistance. It was a reaction against the authority of an Establishment represented by parents, teachers, and authority in general. A decade later, this trend had reversed itself. Then drug use was based on curiosity and social context. Decisions to use were influenced by friends but we noticed a decreased association between non-users and users. This, too, might be indicative of the development of a drug sub-culture in South Africa.

There was, however, no clear prototype of a drug user. Students would not label users as physically inactive or mentally degenerative, but there was an overall negative evaluation of drug users. The reason for this might have been the dangers involved in the use of mind altering substances. The two concerns which clearly stood out in this context were danger of health impairment and fear of addiction.

In the view of most high school seniors, drug users should be treated or rehabilitated. The implication was that regular drug users have something wrong with them and for this reason need treatment or, since they do not have control over their actions, rehabilitation. Black students were clearly not in agreement with treatment or rehabilitation.

As had been the case in earlier discussions, we noticed again a great deal of similarity in the conservative views expressed by Black high school seniors and their counterparts in the Afrikaans medium school. This coincided with the recognition of authority in the parental home—especially with the mother—and with religiosity and social networking.

7

USE OF OTHER DRUGS

Introduction

There was a slight difference in the questionnaires administered to students in 1974 and 1985. In the latter study we essentially duplicated all the questions pertaining to cannabis and applied them to alcohol. The net result of this expansion was that we had much greater volume and greater detail about alcohol use by high school seniors for 1985 than for a decade earlier. This will be reflected in the discussion which follows.

At the end of the questionnaire in both years, a section was included which dealt with other drugs. In the 1974 study this was also the only place in which information pertaining to alcohol was gathered. With reference to these "other drugs," we asked if the student had used any of them, what his or her attitude was to using such drugs, and whether they intended to use them in the future. Bravado might have been an issue if the study had been conducted in person, but the anonymous format mitigated against much misrepresentation in this regard.

Alcohol

In the 1974 questionnaire, we differentiated between beer and wine on the one hand, and spirits on the other. The decision to make such an arbitrary distinction was based on the popularity and availability of African beer, usually the product of simple fermentation of wheat or brown bread. Alcohol content varies from about 2 percent in African beer, 8 percent in commercial bottled beer, between 12 and 20 percent in wine, to near proof in cane spirits. Blacks traditionally used fermented drinks of which *tshwala* was the most common. It has a very low alcohol content

128

and is highly nutritious. In recent years local authorities of Black administration in the urban areas have started to brew an imitation of this beer commercially. In 1985 in urban residential areas Blacks were prohibited from brewing their own beer—not that this has prevented them from doing so—and they were expected to purchase the commercially brewed *ijuba*, known also as KB (Corporation Beer), and by more descriptive terms. Ijuba could be purchased in almost any bottle store in Durban, and its sale is not legally restricted to Blacks. Yet the use of African beer was almost exclusively limited to Blacks. It was considered a traditional drink that quenched their thirst, has vitamins (*linomsoco*) and cools one off. One middle-aged respondent, in related research said that drinking traditional beer was like drinking water: only with the latter you stayed home but with the former you got to socialize.

Many Black workers had ijuba for lunch or stopped by the canteen for a drink after work. The worker who had some of the thick brew after lunch said he also enjoyed it to wash down the meal. Using the same idiom, the worker who stopped off for a can of beer on his way home said "it [was] taken as a wash down after work."

In a previous publication (du Toit 1976), it was pointed out that Blacks in South Africa differed quite markedly in their drinking patterns when compared to the other ethnic groups. Blacks were really the only people who drank ijuba or variations of it; they drank very little wine, for which the urban Blacks had no taste; liquor was increasing in popularity and was becoming associated with sophistication and modernity. With this changing pattern of alcohol use, we should keep in mind that until the early sixties Blacks in South Africa could not purchase alcohol freely. The alcoholic content of the traditionally brewed beer, according to Act 30 of 1928, was limited to 2 percent by volume. In time the government appointed a commission of inquiry, and their positive report resulted in Act 72 of 1961 which permitted Blacks to buy alcoholic beverages freely.

The last thorough study of the drinking patterns of Blacks (Miles 1964) showed the same preferences we have established. Four-fifths of the subjects in this study justified their use of African beer on physiological grounds. In a study comparing rural and urban Blacks, the conclusion was reached that the urban-oriented and urban-committed Blacks were likely to drink commercial beers and liquor and the rural Blacks more likely to use African beer. As education and literacy increased, so did the use of alcoholic beverages of all kinds, and when the subject was urban and well-educated, the preference was toward greater quantities of liquor.

In addition to these kinds of alcoholic beverages, there were a variety of concoctions, most of which were high in alcoholic content and unhealthful due to impurity. Such names as *Skokiaan*, *babaton*, *mfulamfula*, *isiqataviki* (kill-me-quick), and *isishimevani* are familiar to researchers in urban South Africa and more recently *gavini* has been added to the list. These concoctions normally are purchased only by members of the lowest socioeconomic class. In a study of drinking patterns among Blacks in the Durban area, Craig found that sixteen persons or 32 percent of patients at the Kwasimami ("place of recovery and growth") out-patient clinic for Black alcoholics preferred such concoctions. Only two persons or 4.5 percent of her control group preferred these potions with high alcoholic content (1970:76). The reverse was also true in that only 22 percent of the patients preferred African beer, while it was the favorite of 80 percent of the control sample drawn at random. Some of these distilled home brews are referred to as *maconsane*, literally "that which drips." Whole wheat brown bread, *ntombo*-corn, and yeast are the basic ingredients, but some of the more volatile concoctions have been made with potato peels or anything else that will ferment. These concoctions are prepared in secret at private homes or sold in some of the less sophisticated *shebeens*.

In the past, when alcohol use was illegal under most conditions, these drinks had to be consumed in a very short time. Speaking about living conditions in a Black urban slum yard some years ago, Ellen Hellmann remarked:

> Drunkenness is alarmingly prevalent in Rooiyard. The reason is largely to be found in the necessity for drinking quickly, as the danger of detection by the police is ever present. The otherwise comparatively innocuous mqombothi soon makes its effects notice-able if it is drunk quickly instead of being imbibed slowly and at leisure, as was the custom under tribal conditions. Drinks such as skokiaan and shimeya are extremely intoxicating; the effects of isiqataviki it is

claimed, occasionally with pride, often last three days. (1969:92)

The importance of the shebeen and home brew decreased significantly since 1961. Those who drank only African beer mostly bought from Black women who sold in their own homes. Once a day large trucks arrived at various places in the satellite city, and women who were queuing are allowed four gallons per person. It was possible of course to return again or have relatives stand in line on your behalf. On one occasion we saw a queue extending more than seventy yards from the truck. One woman left with thirty gallons of "KB"—the commercially brewed African beer. This beer may simply be sold in the yard or home or may be offered in a shebeen-setting.

Speaking of her research in KwaMashu, a Black satellite city north of Durban where many of our Black students lived, Keirn stated as follows:

Another extra-legal way of earning [money] is to set up a shebeen. Women who pursue this means of augmenting or earning their income convert their lounge into the sitting and drinking area where European liquor and beer may be purchased by the drink and consumed in the company of other men. The proprietress or 'shebeen queen' dispenses beverages from their hiding place in the bedroom and keeps her account book there for her credit customers to sign. Because of the public nature of the shebeen and the danger of police informers among customers, elaborate precautions are taken to protect against raids. The 'shebeen queen' must appraise herself of the evidence required in order for her to be convicted in court and then minimize the chances of such evidence being obtained. While some liquor supplies are purchased at the KwaMashu bottle store, another method of obtaining supplies after the closing of the bottle store or on Sunday, a busy day, is to send someone (a child or another woman) to a particular house at a nearby section where liquor is stored in quantity by a 'wholesaler.' This wholesaler, always

131

referred to by his nickname, sells only by the bottle and has several unofficial outlets in KwaMashu. He is widely successful and his name is heard on visits to other townships near Durban. Both the 'shebeen queens' with whom I was able to become acquainted knew of the 'wholesaler' and used his outlets more or less regularly. Both of these women began their careers in a similar fashion—they needed extra money and having small children to care for at home they did not want to take outside employment. One has since divorced her husband, and the other has already instituted proceedings against her husband. Data collected over the period of one month on the quantities of liquor and beer purchased, the prices paid by the 'shebeen queen,' and the sale price per unit reveal that even the smaller shebeen earns its proprietress R50.00 per month profit. (1970:98-99)

The majority of persons, however, employed a variety of means of acquiring alcohol and used all of these methods. The normal pattern was to have commercially brewed beer or some liquor daily during the week, but to imbibe more than this on weekends. This was the time to visit or to have friends over and to open some "hot stuff" like vodka, gin, whiskey, or brandy. On occasions we saw people in shebeens drink mixtures such as gin-in-beer or vodka-in-beer.

Among students, however, alcohol use is obviously much lower than among adults. Students were asked how many times they had used alcohol—differentiating in 1974 between beer and wine when compared to spirits. But in 1985 the section asked generally about alcohol use and included three questions which differentiated between beer (including tshwala), wine, and liquor.

In 1974 Blacks had the lowest reported incidence of alcohol use with 53.7 percent claiming nonuse. This position was reaffirmed a decade later when 70.6 percent stated that they had not used alcohol. In every other case alcohol use increased: among the Coloured, nonusers declined from 28.7 percent to 18.9 percent of the students; and among White, non-users declined from 11.7 percent to 4.9 percent.

Because of the religious and moral rules of abstention, Indian students must be discussed separately. In the earlier survey, 56.7 percent stated they had never used alcohol. This figure was affected by secularization; a decade later, 35.8 percent claimed never to have used alcohol. While not all Indians are strictly religious or abide by the moral prescriptions of family and tradition, it will be recalled that most of these high school seniors were Hindus and Muslims. Whereas many Hindu rituals recognized cannabis, this did not apply to alcohol. The Koran explicitly forbids the use of alcohol, and we would expect not to find persons who have even experimented with it in this category.

Turning to the White schools, we again found a significant drop in the number of students who had never used alcohol. Seniors in the coeducational school on the city outskirts had 8.8 percent who did not use in 1974; in 1985 that figure was fairly similar at 8.3 percent. The boys' and girls' English medium school both showed a sharp decline respectively from 6.1 percent and 6.4 percent in 1974 to 1.1 percent and 2.8 percent. In a dramatic change the Afrikaans medium school in downtown Durban showed that though 39.7 percent of the seniors in 1974 claimed never to have used alcohol, only 6.1 percent of the seniors a decade later made this claim.

The following discussion refers to the 1985 data since the new section of the questionnaire presented a great deal of data specifically dealing with alcohol use. The previous paragraph presented figures pertaining to students who stated that they had never used alcohol. In a later section of this questionnaire, they were asked about the use of various kinds of alcohol. Here the figures for "never used" differed somewhat from the previous claim. Table 29 presents figures for frequency of use of beer, wine, and liquor respectively. Readers are reminded that in contrast with American "light" beers, the South African beer has an alcohol content of 8 percent by volume and is relatively expensive compared to wine. South Africa is known for its wine production, and many homes use wine on a daily basis. Those who prefer to drink in other settings can buy a bottle of good wine at a price slightly higher than two or three beers would cost. This fact spoke for itself when we noticed that the figure of "never used" was lowest for wine in all four of the ethnic groups. The range of those who claimed nonuse of beer, wine, and liquor, respectively,

133

Table 29
FREQUENCY OF ALCOHOL USE BY HIGH SCHOOL SENIORS IN DURBAN IN 1985

Frequency	Black Beer		Black Wine		Black Liquor		Coloured Beer		Coloured Wine		Coloured Liquor	
	No.	%	No.	%	No.	%	No.	%	No.	%	No.	%
Never	95	75.4	88	69.8	100	79.4	70	38.9	55	30.6	89	49.5
Daily or more	1	0.8	2	1.6	5	4.0	1	0.6	-	-	1	0.6
Once a week or more	10	7.9	3	2.4	6	4.8	15	8.3	3	1.7	8	4.4
1–3 monthly	4	3.2	3	2.4	1	0.8	30	16.7	17	9.4	18	10.0
Every 2–3 months	2	1.6	1	0.8	2	1.6	17	9.4	28	15.6	23	12.8
2–3 times year	3	2.4	7	5.6	6	4.8	20	11.1	34	18.9	17	9.4
Once or less a year	11	8.7	22	17.5	6	4.8	27	15.0	43	23.9	24	13.3
Total	126	100.0	126	100.1	126	100.2	180	100.0	180	100.1	180	100.0

Frequency	Indian Beer		Indian Wine		Indian Liquor		White Beer		White Wine		White Liquor	
	No.	%	No.	%	No.	%	No.	%	No.	%	No.	%
Never	196	57.5	162	47.5	213	62.5	119	28.9	64	15.5	94	22.8
Daily or more	5	1.5			2	0.6	1	0.2	5	1.2	3	0.7
Once a week or more	18	5.3	4	1.2	12	3.5	71	17.2	42	10.2	61	14.8
1–3 monthly	22	6.4	10	2.9	20	5.9	84	20.4	78	18.9	77	18.7
Every 2–3 months	21	6.2	16	4.7	26	7.6	41	10.0	77	18.7	69	16.7
2–3 times year	30	8.8	42	12.3	20	5.9	34	8.3	79	19.2	45	10.9
Once or less a year	49	14.4	107	31.4	48	14.1	62	15.0	67	16.3	63	15.3
Total	341	100.1	341	100.0	341	100.1	412	100.0	412	100.0	412	99.9

was smallest among Blacks, confirming that most Blacks claimed not to have had a palate for wine. As one might expect, the frequency of use was highest among White students, whose economic status, parental home environment, and "sophistication" were deciding factors.

When we compared the four White high schools, the difference in drinking behavior between the English medium and Afrikaans medium schools was obvious. The 1974 findings showed that while 73 percent of the Afrikaans students had never used spirits, the average percentage of students at the two major English schools who abstained was 25 percent. These figures changed in 1985. The ratio of users to nonusers had completely reversed among Afrikaans students in the ten year period. There also had been an increase among the English speaking categories. Table 30 presents the frequency of use of spirits by students in the four White high schools. The conservative position of the Afrikaans medium school is again clear. The seniors in the English boy's school remained the most frequent users—matched by the smallest number who had only experimented or used liquor once a year or less frequently.

Tobacco

Cigarette packages in the United States carry a warning that smoking may be "hazardous to your health," but this warning is omitted in South Africa. Although the workplace and public venues in the United States are increasingly becoming "smoke-free" due to consciousness raising lobbies and educational programs, South Africans happily puff away. The result is a country where smoking is very common, and those in high school regard the use of cigarettes as "cool" and sophisticated. The outsider who visits South Africa is immediately struck by three things: the number of young people who smoke; the number of women who smoke; and the way people smoke—a style I call *aggressive smoking* with little concern for the nonsmoker.

In 1974 we found that Whites constituted the group with the highest percentage of smokers, 70.1 percent. Coloured were second with 55.8 percent and Indian students third as only 45.7 percent of them claimed to have smoked. Black students had the lowest percentage (36.7 percent) of smokers in 1974 and again in

Table 30
FREQUENCY OF USE OF LIQUOR (SPIRITS) BY HIGH SCHOOL SENIORS
IN WHITE HIGH SCHOOLS IN DURBAN IN 1985

Frequency	English Medium High School on City Outskirts		Afrikaans Medium Urban High School		English Medium Wealthy Neighborhood Boys School		English Medium Wealthy Neighborhood Girls School	
	Number	Percent	Number	Percent	Number	Percent	Number	Percent
Never	28	21.2	30	36.6	13	14.4	23	21.3
Daily +	2	1.5	0	0.0	1	1.1	0	0.0
Once weekly +	17	12.9	5	6.1	26	28.9	13	12.0
1-3 a month	26	19.7	9	11.0	14	15.6	28	25.9
Every 2-3 mos.	25	18.9	10	12.2	18	20.0	16	14.8
2-3 a year	15	11.4	8	9.8	10	11.1	12	11.1
Once a year	19	14.4	20	24.4	8	8.9	16	14.8
Total	132	100.0	82	100.0	90	100.0	108	100.0

136

1985. Only 14.3 percent claimed to have smoked. There was quite a drop in 1985 among White high school seniors, 51.9 percent of whom claim to have smoked. The Coloured (at 52.2 percent) and Indian (at 42.8 percent) high school seniors seemed to smoke as much as their predecessors a decade ago. Regular smoking did seem to be decreasing among students. In 1974 36.7 percent of the Indian and 19.0 percent of the Black students were regular smokers. These figures, a decade later, were 24.5 percent and 6.3 percent, respectively.

The position among the different White schools in 1974 was exactly as one would expect it: only 39.0 percent of the Afrikaans students as compared with 79.0 percent (boys' school) and 72.0 percent (girls' school) at the English medium schools. There was, however, an interesting trend: the Afrikaans medium school still showed the same relative percentage (40.2 percent) of students who smoked, the English girls' school in 1985 had 59.3 percent, and the English boys' school had 68.9 percent of the students smoking. The English medium school on the city outskirts remained between these two extremes.

Other drugs

Among other mind-altering practices by students, either on an experimental basis or regularly, most frequently mentioned was "whiffers," or the sniffing of gasses. The use of inhalants was much more common among South African school children than the use of hard drugs. Tetrachloride, cleaning fluids, benzine, and methylated spirits could be found in most kitchens. All a person needed to do to obtain lighter fluid, gasoline, or kerosene was to visit his father's storage room or garage. Around the home, somewhere, he was bound to find paint thinner, shellac, plastic cement, or model airplane glue. The voluntary inhalation or sniffing of volatile organic solvents and compounds was as easy as picking up a cigarette. Allen (1966) and Prebble and Laury (1967) wrote the first reports on this phenomenon in the United States, but not much has been done since then. In spite of the inherent dangers and potential dependence, researchers have concentrated on more exotic drugs instead of the very common, always available supply of hydrocarbons, ketones, alcohols, and glycols. Table 31

Table 31
FREQUENCY OF USE OF INHALANTS BY
HIGH SCHOOL SENIORS IN DURBAN

	Black				Coloured				Indian				White			
	1974		1985		1974		1985		1974		1985		1974		1985	
Frequency	No.	%	No.	%	No.	%	No.	%	No.	%	No.	%	No.	%	No.	%
Never	166	83.4	124	98.4	70	87.5	157	87.2	287	90.3	303	88.9	394	88.6	315	76.5
1-2 times	17	8.5	2	1.6	8	10.0	18	10.0	21	6.6	33	9.7	32	8.1	64	15.5
3-5 times	6	3.0	0	0.0	1	1.2	3	1.7	5	1.6	4	1.2	3	0.8	15	3.6
6-9 times	3	1.5	0	0.0	0	0.0	0	0.0	2	0.6	0	0.0	1	0.3	9	2.2
10+ times	6	3.0	0	0.0	1	1.2	2	1.1	2	0.6	1	0.3	8	2.0	9	2.2
Yes NFI	1	0.5							1	0.3			1	0.3		
Total	199	99.9	126	100.0	80	99.9	180	100.0	318	100.0	341	100.1	439	100.1	412	100.0
No response	29				9				19				59			

indicates that inhalants were a fairly frequently used drug, either on an experimental or regular basis.

Because inhalants appeared to be innoxious, a large number of young persons experiment with them. In 1974, 2 percent of the Whites and 3 percent of the Africans had used these drugs more than ten times or were regular users. We do not have a breakdown by sex, but the two White schools which were segregated by sex showed that the only seven girls who had tried inhalants did so once or twice only; the boys reflect a large number of persons in the once-or-twice category, and six persons in the ten times or more category. The 1985 figures showed a large decrease in the use of inhalants by Black students. Only 1.6 percent of the Blacks said they had ever used them. However, 1.4 percent more Indian students used inhalants in 1985 than in 1974. The number of Coloured students remained the same. There also was an increase in use among White students. In 1974 the Indians had the smallest percentage of experimenters in this category of drug use while the Africans had the highest percentage. The "use of benzine or petrol" was a common categorization by youngsters of their use of inhalants.

The relative picture changed quite dramatically in a decade. Black students seemed to have turned away from sniffing. The percentage of Coloured and Indian students had remained very much the same for those who had used this mind altering method. The most dramatic change could be found among the White students. Here we found an increase from 11.4 percent to 23.5 percent of students who had sniffed some gas.

Turning to a closer look at the White schools to find a reason for the dramatic increase, we saw that it occurred essentially among the seniors at the English medium boys' high school. Of these students, 53.3 percent claimed to have engaged in sniffing. Percentages decrease progressively from the girls' high (20.4 percent), the school on the city outskirts (14.4 percent), to the Afrikaans medium school (9.8 percent).

The next most frequently used mind altering substances were hallucinogens. Relatively few students had used such drugs in 1974 and the relative picture remained the same a decade later. Percentages for 1985 appear in parentheses. In the first drug survey the Black students showed the highest frequency of use at 5.0 percent (.8 percent); Indian high school seniors were next with

3.5 percent (1.2 percent); Whites followed with 1.8 percent (1.9 percent); and Coloureds were close to them with 1.7 percent (1.3 percent). Looking at the figures in parentheses, we see that only the Whites increased their use in the intervening decade. Blacks represented the most dramatic drop.

Amphetamines, which include a variety of "pep pills," were not in great demand. Examples of drugs in the South African context considered to be amphetamines were mentioned in parentheses in the questionnaire so that the students knew what was being discussed. Few South African students claimed to have used this variety of drug. In 1974 only 2.0 percent of the Black respondents, 2.4 percent of the Coloureds, 4.7 percent of the Indians, and 7.7 percent of the Whites had ever used amphetamines. In 1985 there was a dramatic decrease among the first three ethnic groups. No Black student claimed use of this drug; only .6 percent of the Coloureds and 1.2 percent of the Indians did. In the four White high schools, matters had not changed much: 6.4 percent of the students had used amphetamines. The relative distribution of these students conformed to the pattern already discerned. The largest percentage attended English boys' high and the smallest percentage was from the Afrikaans school.

The only other drug with a substantial group of student users was laughing gas. This is a drug which we added to the 1985 survey. Only one Coloured student claimed to have used it, as did 5.8 percent of the Whites.

As was the case with other drug categories, barbiturates were identified by a number of common referents so that the high school seniors knew to what they were responding. In 1974 Whites constituted the smallest number of users, in 1985 the largest. In both cases, though, the total number of persons involved is insignificant. A handful of students had experimented with opium, cocaine, and PCP; but their numbers do not justify discussion. No student in the 1985 sample claimed use of heroin.

Summary

The discussion of other drug use is perhaps the least interesting, though potentially the most important. In cases of multiple drug use or if a drug subculture had developed, it would have been significant. In the case of South African high school students, we found essentially the use of a legal drug present in most homes and used by most parents, and the use of an illegal drug, grown locally and readily available. Black students' claim of nonuse of alcohol contrasted them with the other ethnic groups. Afrikaans students showed a dramatic increase in users but still represented a conservative trend, especially with regard to the use of liquor. Smoking was so common as to be an expected behavior. Blacks and Afrikaans-speaking Whites showed lowest use. In both cases the status of women was a more traditional one, and we would have expected lower use among these female students than among the English-speaking girls.

Van der Burgh (1975), despite the title of his report, *Drugs and South African Youth*, studied a large sample of White males only 16 to 21 years of age, all of whom had left school. They were not quite comparable to our sample of high school seniors of different ethnic group membership, but did provide a frame of reference. Table 32, reproduced here from van der Burgh's study, allowed a comparison, particularly with those who had recently left school. We noticed that in the mid-1970s when both studies were conducted, there was not much difference in the use of other illicit drugs. The figures for cannabis use were lower than our own 1974 study and approximated more closely the figures for the Afrikaans-speaking sample. It was interesting to note that the van der Burgh study sample consisted of 58 percent who spoke Afrikaans at home and only 37 percent who spoke English (the rest were bilingual or spoke other languages, perhaps indicating recent immigrants). The author concluded as follows:

> The percentages do, however, show that in the majority of cases drug use took place after the respondents had already left school yet it is unlikely that the very fact of school-leaving had precipitated this. In all probability this drug use was a continuation of a pattern of behavior that had its origins in the school years. To the extent that there was change, it would seem as if it was mostly in the direction of increasing the use of a particular drug. (1975:15)

Table 32

DAGGA AND OTHER DRUG USE PATTERNS IN THE TWELVE MONTH PERIOD IMMEDIATELY PRIOR TO THE STUDY IN TERMS OF THE PERIOD ELAPSED BETWEEN THE TIME OF LEAVING SCHOOL AND THE TIME OF THE STUDY

Drug use patterns	Period elapsed					Total
	Less than 3 mos.	3-6 mos.	7-11 mos.	1 year-1 year 11 mos.	2 years or more	
	Percentage					
Dagga						
Non-user	90.5	83.5	86.3	81.6	80.3	85.3
Experimental user	3.0	5.9	5.9	7.7	5.4	5.4
Occasional user	3.8	6.1	3.5	4.9	6.4	4.7
Regular user	2.7	4.5	4.3	5.9	8.0	4.7
Total***	100.0	100.0	100.0	100.0	100.0	100.0
N	1,525	559	658	1,253	578	4,573*
Other drugs						
Non-user	97.8	97.7	97.4	95.7	92.4	96.5
Experimental user	1.0	1.2	1.1	1.9	1.6	1.4
Occasional user	0.9	0.7	1.2	1.7	3.5	1.4
Regular user	0.3	0.4	0.3	0.7	2.6	0.7
Total	100.0	100.0	100.0	100.0	100.0	100.0
N	1,525	558	658	1,255	578	4,574**

*   Only 4,573 questionnaires could be used for this cross-tabulation
**   Only 4,574 questionnaires could be used for this cross-tabulation
***   Due to approximation the percentages do not always total 100.0

Source: van der Burgh, C. 1975. *Drugs and South African Youth*. Human Sciences Research Council. Report No. S-38. Pretoria.

8

CONCLUSION

Two points must be restated here. The first is that this study dealt with students of urban high schools, and almost all the students were urban residents. They may have had varying degrees of rural experiences or networks, kin or friendship, but their immediate interaction occurred with fellow city dwellers. The second is that cannabis in South African was always smoked rather than ingested in some way. Though these urban residents expressed involvement with other drugs and with alcohol, one would find less diversity in the drug panorama in a rural area and also less diversity in the drug paraphernalia.

Historical evidence suggests that *Cannabis sativa* has been smoked for at least six centuries in Africa, and we can presume that the ancestors of the Zulu used the drug this way. The ancestors of the Indian students took cannabis in liquid form or mixed it with sweet meats (and even formed a product consisting of cannabis and opium). It is clear that shortly after their arrival in Natal they adopted the method of smoking practiced by the indigenous Black population. They made local adaptations of the water pipe or hubble-bubble whose water container consisted of a dried gourd, an antelope horn or some other object through which the smoke could be passed.

Older Blacks in both rural and urban areas still preferred the traditional horn waterpipe, but it was clumsy and easy to detect during a police raid. Numerous varieties of waterpipes had been innovated, and the sources of construction materials border on the ingenious (du Toit 1980[b]:29-51). Varieties of construction bricks, metal pipes, milk bottles, coconut shells, broken bottle necks, and pop cans had been used in an attempt to imitate the traditional pipe. I suggest there was more involved than simply conscious imitation of form; the process of drawing the smoke through water

143

and thus cooling it down was an added reason, making the activity both imitative and innovative at the same time.

Younger Blacks, and especially those in urban areas where police informers, plain clothed policemen, and police raids were always a possibility, had dispensed with the cumbersome and incriminating pipe and used a variety of cigar or cigarette forms to smoke cannabis. In many cases they may use a regular tobacco smoking pipe or clay chillum filled with pure or mixed cannabis. These new conditions, especially the fear aspect, had not only influenced the mechanism for smoking but also the method of smoking. Absent from the city or town environment is the leisurely "sun-downer" because those who work seldom get home before dark and because of the heterogeneous settlement pattern in which a neighbor might be a police informer. The result was that when smoking was done, it was done in a hurry. A man might take his morning and evening smoke while hiding in his latrine, or his daytime smoke at work during a tea or lunch break. The best place where one was least likely to be discovered was in the open or under a culvert. In such places it was easy to dispose of a broken bottleneck pipe, a cannabis cigarette butt, and any other evidence. The air was clear and the incriminating smell of cannabis drifted away on the light breeze.

Much the same situation applied to the other ethnic groups. During the research one young fellow explained "Boy, the police really hate dagga!" That was true, and the user, irrespective of his status or ethnic group, was a prime target for the special drug squad.

The age of the high school students presented a clear reflection of the South African social structure. Generally speaking Whites had better socioeconomic, domestic, and residential conditions which allowed children to enter school at an early age and to attend regularly, thus matriculating at the expected age of eighteen. Blacks were normally worse off in all these respects and their matriculation age reflected this. Student age also was indicative of primary and secondary school facilities, of the job and part-time job situation, and related factors. Among Whites the total student population was between ages of sixteen and twenty, with 50.7 percent seventeen years of age. One could then expect that the majority of Whites would graduate "on time." This was an anticipated event based on a school starting age of six years and a curriculum spanning twelve years. Indian and Coloured students were very similar and more like the White in their age profile. No White student and only two Coloured and Indian students were over age twenty; fully thirty (23.7 percent) of the Black students were. The implications of such an age disparity were obvious in a number of areas including sexuality (du Toit 1987), role modeling, drug use, and it would seem, wisdom about drugs which may have a physical or legal implication for personal improvement.

Religion was an important factor which should be emphasized when comparing the subcategories of the White group. Whites in this study represented two groups; an essentially English-speaking group and an Afrikaans-speaking group. Among the former, those who did not reside in the wealthy neighborhood showed greater religious diversity, but the boys' and girls' school students paralleled each other almost perfectly. The group in which the greatest uniformity was found was in the Afrikaans school. Here we found 76.8 percent of all the senior students belonging to the Dutch Reformed Church. This was a very conservative church from a strong Calvinist tradition. There was an emphasis on Biblical prescription, or "the decent way of behaving," and coupled to this was strong family tradition and recognition of paternal authority.

The solidarity of the family was a clear reflection of the conservative and religious emphasis of society. The lowest separation and divorce rates were found among Indians and Afrikaners. In both of these categories, one could expect a greater likelihood of one parent being home. Bachman et al. (1981:63) noted that students who were not living with both parents were more likely to use cannabis. Our own findings regarding both cannabis and alcohol use among American students confirmed this (du Toit and Suggs 1985; Suggs and du Toit 1985).

If the reader keeps in mind the South African color caste system in which members of political minority groups, but especially Blacks, must use everything at their disposal to improve themselves, the significance of future plans gains in importance. In 1985 by far the majority of Blacks wanted to get away from the uncertainty of unskilled jobs, and almost 73 percent planned to go to university or college. This figure was higher than a decade previously and was almost double the figure for any other ethnic group. A further 20 percent planned to attend a technicon, where they could learn a skill and qualify for a job giving predictability and a fair income. The other ethnic groups were fairly similar in terms of their future plans.

The economic background of the family may have influenced the likelihood of using certain kinds of drugs. Frequently, as was the case with White students, those at high income English medium schools were more likely to have parents who would have been tolerant of experimentation with drugs. These students may also have had enough money to acquire such substances. It was not strange to find that Whites had the highest percentage of parents in managerial and professional occupations, while Blacks not only had the lowest percentage of parents in these occupations but also the smallest range of jobs available.

We should be hesitant in a culturally and ethnically heterogeneous society such as existed in South Africa to ascribe drug use, and particularly cannabis smoking, to an economic cause, or any single cause. We must consider traditions which are historically and culturally derived. There is no simplistic answer.

For a long time it was maintained in South Africa that Blacks used cannabis because it was inexpensive. Since the Blacks were at the lowest level of the economic scale the argument goes that they would use cheap alcohol and cannabis rather than the more expensive substances. For some time I have argued for consideration of sociocultural reasons. The material presented here leans convincingly in the direction of long standing traditions of cannabis use as well as the use of tshwala, the Zulu home brewed beer. These are cultural-historical rather than economic reasons. Much the same argument could be presented for the Indian subjects in our sample. The Indians in Natal are financially fairly well off. We find here strong continuities of ritual, medicinal, and contextual uses of drugs. These involve mostly the continued value placed on cannabis in certain contexts and the method of use (that is with the chillum). Nevertheless, some changes have occurred through acculturation. The Indians of South Africa have assumed local referents, they have borrowed the use of various hubble-bubbles from Blacks, and follow much the same method of firing and smoking cannabis.

When we considered the use of cannabis, we found about the same relative percentages of users among Whites and Blacks at high school in 1974. In the 1985 survey, fewer Blacks admitted to

146

cannabis use; more Coloureds and Whites did, and the same percentage of Indians did, making the latter three groups almost identical.

Living conditions in the Black ghettos contrasted quite starkly with the luxury of some of the affluent White neighborhoods. In the Black household children may have been left to their own devices during the day because parents were working; in the White neighborhood children also were left frequently to their own devices when the father worked and the mother may have been out on social or sporting activities. Parental supervision did influence drug use, particularly experimentation and first use. In the 1985 survey, we found that most Black students started using cannabis before and during junior high school. This contrasted with all the other groups in which first use generally occurred during their senior high school years.

Looking at bonds of amity, we found that peer group age mates rather than older siblings or kinsmen usually introduced users to the drug. High school students, however, did not smoke at school nor were their school friends the most active cannabis smokers. The importance of the peer group has been demonstrated in a variety of drug-using contexts. Winick (1965) emphasized that smoking cannabis was a social activity and the importance of sharing with other young people.

Questions dealing with alcohol use of both parents and respondents reflected a number of aspects that must be addressed. Among White and Coloured (and some Blacks), alcohol use reflected the respondents' economic position. This implied both the ability to purchase beverages as well as their availability in the parental home. Indians (particularly women) used less alcohol; for Muslims, there are severe, negative injunctions in the Koran. These questions also represented what might be interpreted as a slight oversight on our part for not differentiating specifically between tshwala, and the commercial bottled variety of beer. It will be recalled that Blacks in this region traditionally used fermented drinks as was common throughout Africa (Pan 1975). The alcoholic content of such brews was low and the beers highly nutritious and "good for you" (Curtis 1973). While nutritional value was unlikely to be the deciding factor in tshwala use, its traditional value was. On numerous occasions this writer had visited educated and even professional Blacks in South Africa and

147

been invited to share in a late afternoon "wash down." In some cases the traditional *kamba*, black clay pot, would be used, in others a tall glass.

We examined the association between the use of alcohol and cannabis by parents and their attitudes regarding experimentation and use by their children. We found that the most lenient views were expressed by the parents of White children; the most conservative views were held by the parents of Black students.

The same ethnic differentiation emerged from questions about the orientation of students. African and Afrikaans students were very strongly parent oriented, whereas the English-speaking White students were peer group oriented. In both the latter categories, teachers figured strongly. But when we asked for the reasons why these young people tried or used cannabis, the picture of peer pressure reemerged. Most of the students stated that they were inquisitive or they did it for kicks. More than 12 percent of the White students, and particularly girls at a posh English medium high school, saw cannabis use as a symbol of resistance! In the 1985 survey we noticed an absence of the intergenerational conflict which grew out of the "sixties syndrome." In 1985 most of the students used cannabis for kicks or to feel good.

The use or nonuse of various substances is frequently influenced by the amount of knowledge available concerning their effects. Thus folk beliefs about the danger of a foodstuff might lead to its disappearance from the market. But an absence of such beliefs, which are based on folk models or empirical studies, may lead to the popularization of a highly dangerous practice such as sniffing and inhalation of benzine and other toxic solvents. The question arises, then, why certain young people smoked cannabis and others avoided the drug. Among Black students the cannabis smoker was seen as representing the lower class or as being morally degenerate. In part this was due to the large number of unemployed who smoked or the large number of persons who had been arrested and returned from jail as drug users. (Pressure from fellow prisoners was very great and numerous informants ascribed their drug use to a nondrug related arrest and period of incarceration.) Coloured students and in 1985 also Indian and White youths characterized cannabis users as psychological cases who need counseling. In a later question (Table 28), these three categories of respondents recommended that drug users should receive rehabilitation treatment and counseling. Based on knowing persons who used the drug, most students saw little difference in the physical activity level of those who smoked the drug and those who did not.

If students in reality saw little difference between users and non-users, we would expect to find normal acceptance of users as friends, club members, and dating partners. If, on the other hand, they had reservations about the use of the drug, then this too would be reflected in friendships. We found, in fact, that almost three-fourths of all Coloured and Indian students would attempt to persuade a friend to stop smoking the drug. About the same number of Black students would act in this fashion. As before, the Whites would be most accepting of a drug-using friend. In the latter category, however, we found the anomalous situation of the Afrikaans high school students. While the English students were relatively accepting of a drug user, the Afrikaans students influenced the figures for Whites by reacting negatively in almost 88 percent of the cases—the highest of any ethnic group. In the 1985 survey, we found essentially the same position. The Afrikaans students were most critical of drug use by a friend, and the seniors at the White boys' school were most permissive. Both studies showed that, to some degree, the English-speaking White students were willing to disregard drug use. By a wide margin, the Afrikaans students were the group who would be least willing to disregard a friend's cannabis use.

Friendship does not imply gender. Dating, on the other hand, suggests intimacy and the possibility of a lasting relationship with a member of the opposite sex. In the earlier survey we found that a very small percentage of Whites stated that they would not date a person who had tried the drug; Afrikaans-speaking and Black high school seniors responded almost identically. However, among those who stated emphatically that they would not date a person who had tried cannabis, we found almost 50 percent of the Black students and more than 55 percent of the Afrikaans students. The Coloured and Indian students fell midway between these strongly negative views and the more permissive position of the English medium White schools. Having experimented with this drug is not too serious or threatening. But to make things more difficult, the respondents were then asked about *dating a regular*

149

cannabis user. The negative responses here were much more frequent than in the previous case, and even among liberal English-speaking Whites, more than half would not date a regular user. Except for the Blacks who were negative about any person who had used cannabis, in the 1985 sample each of the other three ethnic groups more than doubled the number of negative responses regarding dating a user. It is of interest that almost three out of every four Whites were negative and that in this question, only the Indian students had a higher percentage of negative responses. This would suggest that although persons might have a relatively open mind concerning cannabis use, its implication, and effects, their minds turn conservative when the question of drug use pertains to persons with whom they are very close.

The principle reason for this conservatism and protectionism was the fear that a cannabis smoker would damage his health. This was the first and most frequently mentioned effect among students in all four ethnic groups. That possible effect was mentioned six to eight times as frequently among high school seniors as any other. The next most frequently mentioned risk taken by a cannabis smoker was psychological dependence or addiction. In 1985, possibly due to media attention to this topic, fear of addiction became a major risk as seen by all ethnic groups except the Blacks. A general fear of damage to health remained the primary risk. But the undercurrent of conservatism and concern which we had detected emerged more clearly in responses to a question on appropriate legal control for cannabis use. White and Indian high school students in 1974 clearly preferred the same penalties for cannabis use; Coloured pupils would have liked to see the same penalties joined with increased use of the drug for experimental research. This was the first choice of Blacks. I have suggested that Blacks responded the way they did in part because they had experienced harassment and in part because they must "try harder," but there was still a tradition of cannabis use among them. In 1985 we found that the Black students were the only ones who advocated in any numbers the abolition of legal restrictions. The latter response was the most popular among Blacks while Coloureds, Indians, and Whites would have preferred to see the status quo.

150

At the time of the study in 1974, South Africa did not have a rehabilitation program for cannabis users. We introduced this possibility in the questionnaire. Of the four ethnic group categories of respondents at high school level, three selected rehabilitation as the appropriate punishment for a person found guilty of cannabis smoking. The sole exception were the Black high school seniors. They gave a gut-level response in terms of the threats they hear most frequently. In 44 percent of the cases they stated that a person found guilty should be sent to jail. Their second choice, born of the same prototype, was that such a person should be warned and released. These two responses represented 67.5 percent of Black responses. In 1985 they still did; exactly the same percentage of Black students selected them but in reverse order. In the 1985 survey there was greater support for a warning instead of prosecution. Rehabilitation once again was the reaction preferred by the other three groups.

Turning to the use of other drugs, the former pattern of responses held true. The conservative Afrikaner pupils approximated most closely their Black age mates. The relatively high frequency of alcohol avoidance among Indian students was due to the strong religious undercurrent among Hindus and Moslems alike. This conservatism was present in both the 1974 survey and the 1985 study. Relatively few students used amphetamines, so that comparison between our sample and that of Hindmarch was difficult for a number of reasons. His subjects were predisposed toward amphetamines because "cannabis costs more per unit on the black market than do the amphetamines" (1972:25). There was, of course, quite a difference between South Africa and the United Kingdom. Then, too, he found that 85 percent of the school-aged drug users had used amphetamines. The incidence clearly contrasts with our interethnic sample. There was a greater comparability between our data and the situation in the Netherlands. Buikhuisen and Timmerman concluded that in spite of the fact that between 13 percent and 14 percent of their school sample had tried amphetamines (1972:14), "hashish and marijuana seem to be by far the most popular. The substances were taken by 88.3 percent of the users" (1972:9).

In our 1985 study we included laughing gas as an addition to the category of inhalants. Nitrous oxide usually used as an anesthetic acts on the brain, liver, and other organs. It is much more popular in the U.S., but not widely used in South Africa, possibly due to cost and certainly because of the availability of other inhalants. The inhalation of solvent vapors, unfortunately was much more popular; these could result in headache, nausea, vomiting, skin irritation, as well as more serious effects. Acute intoxication follows the inhalation of hydrocarbons such as are found in benzene, toluene (present in airplane glue), and xylene, especially since the latter two, which could be used in their pure form, are used in cleaners and usually contain amounts of benzene. Lucas (1953:109) pointed out that inhalation of these vapors could result in "salivation, muscular tremors, vomiting, difficult respiration . . . severe cramps and convulsions; fall in body temperature and in blood pressure . . . hemorrhage; deep narcosis and death" (see also Novak et al. 1980).

The problem with inhalants was that they were readily available in household products. Lighter fluid, gasoline, liquid paper, thinner, refrigerant gas, glue, spray paint, finger nail polish remover, cleaning fluids, sealers, spray deodorants, amyl nitrite, toluene, and nitrous oxide are always to be found. With the usual peer influence, low cost, ease of availability, convenient packaging, mood enhancement, nature of the intoxication and absence of legal hassle (Cohen 1978), the inhalant was attractive to youngsters. In the United States the Department of Health and Human Services reviewed the use of hallucinogens and inhalants as a group and warned that continued use of these substances may result in toxicity to the liver, kidneys, and bone marrow, as well as peripheral nerve damage. There also was evidence "for a growing incidence of brain toxicity" (1984:140).

In the U.S., inhalants tended to be used among the younger age group; nitrous oxide among a slightly older group. During the 1970s there was a slight decrease in use among students in the U.S., but then the frequency began to rise again. "For the upper grade levels there has been a continued gradual rise since 1980 in lifetime prevalence, whereas the curves have been more uneven in the lower grades" (Johnston, O'Malley, and Bachman 1986:83). When we used cultural variables as causative factors as we had been doing, other questions arose. Among these were the degree of cultural homogeneity and the tempo of change to which families were subjected. Goldstein (1978) found that among families where an Indian language was used exclusively, there was almost one-third as much use of inhalants as among families where English was spoken. The families that spoke only an Indian language showed less transition and greater stability; the children showed less deviance. The groups in our study which represented the greatest degree of transition and the least stability were Whites and Coloureds, with Indians increasingly becoming less traditional. These sociocultural factors were also reflected in the incidence of drug use—specifically, in this case, the use of inhalants.

In retrospect, drug use by South African students compared favorably with that of other student populations for whom we have data. But this was a temporary phenomenon. The conservative pockets of students comprise Blacks (frequently those with a traditional background), Indians (especially Indian women who were closely tied with traditional religions), and the Afrikaans-speaking component of the White population. In 1985 all three were in a state of rapid change. Blacks were increasingly committing themselves to urban lifestyles and losing some of their rural village ties. Along with this change was the emergence of new values which frequently contradicted traditional behaviors and values. The style of smoking had already changed. Blacks, too, through united opposition groups and a slowly changing political philosophy among the dominant Whites, were acquiring increased human rights with the result that arrest and jail were not as likely to be experienced as they were previously. As Black attitudes changed, these considerations were reflected in a new generation of scholars and students who shared more of a world view with their fellow students of other ethnic backgrounds. The breakdown of the Indian family and increased secularization among youths was already showing its effects. This applied in particular to women for whom secularization and professional aspirations produced a Westernized person who competed with males and was free to use alcohol and to smoke—frequently cannabis. It should be kept in mind also that major inroads had been made among Indians by Pentecostal and other missionizing religions. Oosthuizen (1975) described how this happened in the Durban Indian community, and such changes represented the breakdown not only of traditional religions and values but also of the traditional closed social group. The third group which produced a conservative trend comprised the Afrikaans medium high school seniors. It was possible that persons with this background and

153

tradition may be included among the other "White" categories and that their presence produced a conservative effect there. Increasingly we were finding that the isolationist mentality of the Afrikaner was giving way to interaction and communication not only with Whites of other language groups and philosophies but also with many foreigners—both in South Africa and abroad.

These trends can be summarized. Black students in 1985 seemed to be more conservative than the 1974 cohort group, and there was an increase in the "never used" category. This is quite consistent with other African data (Nevadomsky 1981; 1982). Among Afrikaans students, there was doubling of acceptance and support for users; less differentiation between using versus nonusing classmates; and a significant decrease of those who would disassociate interaction purely on the basis of drug use. In spite of these changes, Afrikaans students were still the most conservative group among the Whites.

Summarizing his study of drug use among White males, van der Burgh concludes as follows:

> While it is clear that an increasing proportion of South
> African youth are presently interested in drugs (and
> will be in the future) the vast majority of the age group
> studied here are still cautious about illicit drugs and
> illicit use of drugs and are not deeply involved in them.
> In a phrase, contemporary South African youth have
> been shown to be less radical (or more traditional)
> than their public image would indicate. On the other
> hand, the striking relationship between the use
> particularly of dagga and a host of other attitudes and
> behaviours, suggests that a great deal more is involved
> here than conformity with a superficial fad. Illicit drug
> use seems to be an integral part of a newly emerging
> life-style. (1975:50)

We would concur with these conclusions but at the high school level at least, other drugs did not seem to play an important role. What we did find, however, was a growing uniformity in patterns of use. Cannabis use was lower among (Black) students, although by traditional influence, we would expect it to be greater But those groups which we expected to be more conservative, such as Indians, showed rapid change. Ethnic isolation was at an end. South African society was emerging as a multihued, multicultural, linguistically diverse mosaic. While I am not suggesting a melting pot, I am suggesting that the pots are so close together that they are affecting the brew which each contains. If this was true in 1974, it was even more so in 1985 as certain legal restrictions were being relaxed and a great deal of interethnic contact was taking place. In 1985 even the aromas from the different brews were blending.

BIBLIOGRAPHY

Ahlstrom-Laakso, S. 1979. *Trends in Drinking Habits Among Finnish Youth from the Beginning of the 1960s to the Late 1970s*. The State Alcohol Monopoly, Social Research Institute of Alcohol Studies, Helsinki. Reports from the Social Research Institute of Alcohol Studies, No. 128.

Alberti, Ludwig. 1968. *Account of the Tribal Life and Customs of the Xhosa in 1807*. Translated by William Fehr. Cape Town: Balkema.

Alexander, C. N., Jr. and E. Q. Campbell. 1967. "Peer Influences on Adolescent Drinking." *Quarterly Journal of Studies on Alcohol* 28.

Anumonye, Amechi. 1980. "Drug Use Among Young People in Lagos, Nigeria." *Bulletin on Narcotics* 32.

Arbousset, T. and F. Daumas. 1846. *Narrative of an Exploratory Tour of the North-East of the Colony of the Cape of Good Hope*. Cape Town: Saul Soloman.

Bachman, Jerald G., et al. 1981. "Smoking, Drinking, and Drug Use Among American High School Students: Correlates and Trends, 1975-1979." *American Journal of Public Health* 71/1.

Baines, Thomas. 1964. *Journal of Residence in Africa 1842-1853*. Vol. 2. R. F. Kennedy (ed.). Cape Town: The Van Riebeeck Society.

Balkisson, B. A. 1973. *A Study of Certain Personality Characteristics of Male, Urban Indians with Drinking Problems*. Unpublished M.Sc. Thesis. University of Natal.

Beauvais, Fred, E. R. Oetting, and R. W. Edwards. 1985. "Trends in Drug Use of Indian Adolescents Living on Reservations: 1975-1983." *American Journal of Drug and Alcohol Abuse* 11.

Bell, D. S., R. A. Champion, and A. J. E. Rowe. 1975. *Monitoring Drug Use in New South Wales: 1971 to 1973.* Sydney: Health Commission of New South Wales.

Bird, John. 1888. *The Annals of Natal 1495-1845*, Vol. 1. Pietermaritzburg: Leonard Bayly.

Blachford, L. 1977. *Summary Report — Surveys of Student Drug Use.* San Mateo, California. Department of Public Health and Welfare.

Bothma, J. H. (ed.). 1951. "Ek was n daggaroker." *Die Brandwag* 15.

Braucht, G. N. 1973. "Deviant Drug Use in Adolescence. A Review of Psychosocial Correlates." *Psychological Bulletin* 76.

————. 1980. "Psychosocial Research on Teenage Drinking: Past and Future." In *Drugs and the Youth Culture* ed. F. R. Scarpitti and S. K. Batesman. Pages 109-43. Beverly Hills, California: Sage Publishers.

Britt, D. W. and E. Q. Campbell. 1977. "A Longitudinal Analysis of Alcohol Use, Environmental Conduciveness and Normative Structure." *Journal of Studies on Alcohol* 38.

Bryant, A. T. 1949. *The Zulu People as They Were Before the White Man Came.* Pietermaritzburg: Shuter & Shooter.

"Butch." 1972. Ek was jare n daggaslaaf. *Oggendblad* 22.

Casalis, E. 1965. *The Basuto or Twenty-three Years in South Africa.* (Originally published in 1861.) Cape Town: C. Struik Pty. Ltd.

Champion R. A., G. J. Egger, and P. Frebilco. 1978. "Monitoring Drug and Alcohol Use and Attitudes Among School Students in New South Wales: 1977 Results." *Australian Journal of Alcohol and Drug Dependence* 5.

Chattopadhyaya, H. P. 1970. *Indians in Africa: A Socioeconomic Study.* Calcutta: Bookland Private Ltd.

Cohen, Sidney. 1978. "Why Solvents?" In *Voluntary Inhalation of Industrial Solvents* ed. Charles Wm. Sharp and L. Thomas Carroll. National Institute on Drug Abuse. Washington, D.C.: U.S. Government Printing Office.

Conder, C. R. 1887. "The Present Condition of the Native Tribes of Bechuanaland." *Journal of the Anthropological Institute* 16.

Craig, Heather Dawn. 1970. *The Drinking Pattern in Kwa Mashu Bantu Township*. Unpublished Masters Thesis, University of Natal, Durban.

Curtis, Donald, 1973. "Cash Brewing in a Rural Economy." *Botswana Notes and Records* 5.

Department of Health and Human Services. 1984. *Drug Abuse and Drug Abuse Research*. Washington, D.C.: U.S. Government Printing Office.

Decle, L. 1898. *Three Years in Savage Africa*. London: Methuen.

Dickie-Clark, H. F. 1966. *The Marginal Situation*. New York: The Humanities Press.

_____. 1972. "The Coloured Minority in Durban." In *The Blending of Races* ed. N. P. Gist and A. G. Dwarkin. New York: Wiley Interscience.

Dishion, Thomas J. and Rolf Loeber. 1985. "Adolescent Marijuana and Alcohol Use: The Role of Parents and Peers Revisited." *American Journal of Drug and Alcohol Abuse* 11.

Dizmang, L. H., J. Watson, P. May, and J. Bopp. 1974. "Adolescent Suicide at an Indian Reservation." *American Journal of Orthopsychiatry* 44.

Downs, William R. 1987. "A Panel Study of Normative Structure, Adolescent Alcohol Use and Peer Alcohol Use." *Journal of Studies on Alcohol* 48.

du Toit, Brian M. 1964. "Substitution, a Process in Culture Change." *Human Organization* 23/1.

_____. 1966. "Color, Class and Caste in South Africa." *Journal of Asian and African Studies* 1/3.

_____. 1974. "Cannabis sativa in Sub-Saharan Africa." *South African Journal of Science* 70/9.

_____. 1975. "Dagga: The History and Ethnographic Setting of Cannabis sativa in Southern Africa." In *Cannabis and Culture* ed. Vera Rubin. The Hague: Mouton.

_____. 1976(a). "Continuity and Change in Cannabis Use by Africans in South Africa." *Journal of Asian and African Studies* 11/3-4.

_____. 1976(b). "Man and Cannabis in Africa: A Study of Diffusion." *African Economic History* 1.

_____. 1977(a). "Historical and Cultural Factors Influencing Drug Use Among Indians in South Africa." *Journal of Psychedelic Drugs* 9/3.

_____. 1977(b). "Ethnicity and Patterning in South African Drug Use." In *Drugs, Rituals, and Altered States of Consciousness* ed. Brian M. du Toit. Rotterdam: Balkema Publishers.

_____. 1980(a). "Linguistic Subterfuge — Its Use by Drug Users in South Africa." *Anthropological Linguistics* 22/1.

_____. 1980(b). *Cannabis in Africa*. Rotterdam: Balkema Publishers.

_____. 1987. "Menarche and Sexuality Among a Sample of Black South African Schoolgirls." *Social Science and Medicine* 24/7.

_____. 1990. *Aging and Menopause Among Indian South African Women*. Albany: State University of New York Press.

du Toit, Brian M., and David N. Suggs. 1985. "Parents, Peers and Pot: Cannabis Use Among High School Students in a Southern County." *Florida Journal of Anthropology*, 10/1.

Editorial. 1958. "Dagga (Cannabis sativa) Smoking in Southern Rhodesia." *The Central African Journal of Medicine* 4.

Ellenberger, D. F., and J. C. MacGregor. 1912. *History of the Basuto, Ancient and Modern*. London: Craxton Publishing Co.

Elphick, Richard. 1977. *Kraal and Castle*. New Haven: Yale University Press.

Ferguson, F. 1968. "Navajo Drinking." *Human Organization* 27.

Fromm, Erich. 1944. "Individual and Social Origins of Neurosis." *American Sociological Review* 9.

Gardiner, Allen F. 1836. *Narrative of a Journey to the Zoolu Country in South Africa Undertaken in 1835*. London: William Crofts.

Godfrey, Peter. 1955. "I Smoked Dagga." *Spotlight* 6.

Goldstein, George S. 1978. "Inhalant Abuse Among the Pueblo Tribes of New Mexico." In *Voluntary Inhalation of Industrial Solvents* ed. Charles Wm. Sharp and L. Thomas Carroll. National Institute on Drug Abuse. Washington, D.C.: U.S. Government Printing Office.

Gomberoff, M., R. Florenzano, and J. Thomas. 1972. "A Study of the Conscious Motivations and the Effects of Marijuana Smoking on a Group of Adolescents in Chile." *Bulletin on Narcotics* 24.

Grout, Lewis. 1970. *Zululand; or Life Among the Zulu-Kafirs of Natal and Zululand, South Africa*. (Originally published in 1861.) London: African Publications Society.

Harley-Mason, R. J. 1938. "The Confessions of a Bhang Smoker." *The East African Medical Journal* 14.

Hartnoll, R., and M. Mitcheson. 1973. "Attitudes of Young People Toward Drug Use." *Bulletin on Narcotics* 25.

Haworth, A. 1982. "A Preliminary Report on Self-Reported Drug Use Among Students in Zambia." *Bulletin on Narcotics* 34.

Hellmann, Ellen. 1969. Rooiyard, A Sociological Survey of an Urban Native Slum Yard. *Rhodes-Livingstone Papers*, Number 13. (Originally published in 1948.) Manchester: Manchester University Press.

Homel, Peter, and Bruce Flaherty. 1986. "Alcohol Use by Australian Secondary School Students." *The Journal of Drug Issues* 16.

Igra, A., and R. H. Moos. 1979. "Alcohol Use Among College Students: Some Competing Hypotheses." *Journal of Youth and Adolescence* 8.

Jensen, G. F., J. H. Stauss, and V. W. Harris. 1977. "Crime, Delinquence, and the American Indian." *Human Organization* 36.

Jessor, R., and S. L. Jessor. 1977. *Problem Behavior and Psychosocial Development: A Longitudinal Study of Youth*. New York: Academic Press.

Johnson, Bruce D. 1973. *Marihuana Users and Drug Subcultures*. New York: John Wiley.

Johnston, Thomas F. 1975. "Dagga Use Among the Shangana-Tsonga of Mozambique and the Northern Transvaal." *Zeitschrift fur Ethnologie* 98.

_____. 1977. "Auditory Driving, Hallucinogens, and Music-Color Synthesia in Tsonga Ritual." In *Drugs, Rituals, and Altered States of Consciousness* ed. Brian M. du Toit. Rotterdam: Balkema.

Johnston, L. D., S. G. Bachman, and P. M. O'Malley. 1984. *Monitoring the Future: Questionnaire Responses from the Nation's High School Seniors, 1983*. Ann Arbor: Institute for Social Research, the University of Michigan.

Johnston, Lloyd D., and Patrick M. O'Malley. 1986. "Why do the Nation's Students Use Drugs and Alcohol? Self-reported

Reasons from Nine National Surveys." *The Journal of Drug Issues* 16.

Johnston, Lloyd D., Patrick M. O'Malley, and Jerald G. Bachman. 1985. *Use of Licit and Illicit Drugs by America's High School Students 1975-1984.* Washington, D.C.: U.S. Government Printer.

_____. 1986. *Drug Use Among American High School Students, College Students, and Other Young Adults.* National Institute on Drug Abuse. Washington, D.C.: U.S. Government Printing Office.

Junod, Henri A. 1927. *The Life of a South African Tribe*, Vol. I. (Originally published in 1912.) London: MacMillan.

Kandel, Denise. 1973. "Adolescent Marihuana Use: Role of Parents and Peers." *Science* 181.

_____. 1975. "Stages in Adolescent Involvement in Drug Use." *Science* 190.

Kandel, Denise, Eric Single, and Ronald C. Kessler. 1976. "The Epidemiology of Drug Use Among New York State High School Students: Distribution, Trends, and Change in Roles of Use." *American Journal of Public Health* 66.

Kandel, Denise, Israel Adler, and Myriano Ludit. 1981. "The Epidemiology of Adolescent Drug Use in France and Israel." *American Journal of Public Health* 71.

Kaplan, H. B., and Pokorny, A. D. 1978. "Alcohol Use and Self-Enhancement Among Adolescents: A Conditional Relationship." In *Currents in Alcoholism.* Vol. 4. Ed. F. A. Seixas. Psychiatric, Psychological, Social and Epidemiological Studies, pp. 51-75. New York: Grune and Stratton.

Keirn, Susan M. 1970. *Roles, Statuses, and Family Life Among Urban African Women.* Unpublished M.A. thesis, University of Florida.

Kolb, Peter. 1968. *The Present State of the Cape of Good Hope.* Vol. I. (Originally published in 1731.) Ed. W. Peter Carstens. London: Johnson Reprint Corporation.

Kondapi. C. 1951. *Indians Overseas 1838-1949.* New Delhi: Indian Council of World Affairs.

Kuper, Hilda. 1960. *Indian People in Natal.* Pietermaritzburg: University of Natal Press.

Latrobe, C. I. 1969. *Journal of a Visit to South Africa in 1815 and 1816.* Cape Town: C. Struik Pty.

161

Levy, Jerrold E., and Stephen J. Kunitz. 1974. *Indian Drinking.* New York: John Wiley.

Lichtenstein, Henry. 1928. *Travels in Southern Africa in the Years 1803, 1804, 1805, and 1806.* Vol. I. (Originally published in 1812.) Translated by Anne Plumtre. Cape Town: The Van Riebeeck Society.

Linton, Ralph. 1936. *The Study of Man.* New York: Appleton-Century Crofts.

Livingstone, David, and Charles. 1865. *Narrative of an Expedition to the Zambesi and its Tributaries.* London: John Murray.

Lucas, G. H. W. 1953. *The Symptoms and Treatment of Acute Poisoning.* New York: MacMillan.

Margulies, R. Z., R. C. Kessler, and D. B. Kandel. 1977. "A Longitudinal Study of Drinking Among High School Students." *Journal of Studies on Alcohol* 38.

Marwick, Brian A. 1940. *The Swazi.* Cambridge: The University Press.

May, P. 1982. "Substance Abuse and American Indians." *International Journal of the Addictions* 17.

McLaughlin, Robert J., Paul E. Baer, Mary A. Burnside, and Alex D. Pokorny. 1985. "Psychosocial Correlates of Alcohol Use at Two Age Levels During Adolescence." *Journal of Studies on Alcohol* 46.

Medicine, B. 1982. "New Roads to Coping: Siouxan Society." In *New Directions in Prevention Among American Indian and Alaska Native Communities* ed. S. Mason. Oregon Health Sciences, University of Portland.

Medina-Mora, M. E., S. Castro, C. Campillo-Serrano, and F. A. Gomez-Mont. 1981. "Validity and Reliability of a High School Drug Use Questionnaire Among Mexican Students." *Bulletin on Narcotics* 33.

Meer, Fatima. 1969. *Portrait of Indian South Africans.* Durban: Premier Press.

Mentzel, O. F. 1944. *A Geographical and Topographical Description of the Cape of Good Hope 1785.* Translated and edited by G. V. Marais and J. Hoge. Cape Town: The Van Riebeeck Society.

Miles, J. D. 1964. *Die Drinkpatroon van die Bantoes in Suid Afrika*. Nasionale Buro vir Opvoedkundige en Maatskaplike Navorsing. Navorsingsreeks, Nr. 18. Pretoria.

Murray, David M., Cheryl L. Perry, Catherine O'Connell and Linda Schmid. 1987. "Seventh-Grade Cigarette, Alcohol, and Marijuana Use: Distribution in a North-Central U.S. Metropolitan Population." *The International Journal of the Addictions* 22.

Nevadomsky, J. 1981. "Patterns of Self-Reported Drug Use Among Secondary School Students in Bendel State, Nigeria." *Bulletin on Narcotics* 33.

_____. 1982. "Self-Reported Drug Use Among Secondary School Students in Two Rapidly Developing Nigerian Towns." *Bulletin on Narcotics* 34.

Nienaber, G. S. 1963. *Hottentots*. Pretoria: J. L. van Schaik.

Novak, Allen, et al. 1980. "The Deliberate Inhalation of Volatile Substances." *Journal of Psychedelic Drugs* 12/2.

Oelting, E. R., and G. S. Goldstein. 1979. "Drug Use Among Native American Adolescents." In *Youth Drug Abuse: Problems, Issues and Treatment*. Toronto: Lexington Books.

O'Neil, Owen Rowe. 1921. *Adventures in Swaziland*. London: George Allen and Unwin.

Oosthuizen, G. C.. 1975. "Pentecostal Penetration into the Indian Community in Metropolitan Durban, South Africa." *Human Sciences Research Council*, Publ. Series No. 52. Durban: Interprint.

Pan, Lynn. 1975. *Alcohol in Colonial Africa*. The Finnish Foundation for Alcohol Studies. Vol. 22. Helsinki.

Pinto, L. J. 1973. "Alcohol and Drug Abuse Among Native American Youth on Reservations: A Growing Crisis." In *Drug Abuse in America: Problems in Perspective*, Vol. 1, pp. 1157-78. Washington, D.C.: Government Printing Office.

Raven-Hart, R. 1971. *Cape Good Hope 1652-1702. The First Fifty Years of Dutch Colonization as Seen by Callers*, Vol. I. Cape Town: Balkema.

Report of the Indian Hemp Drug Commission 1893-94. 1971. (Originally Published in 1894.) New York: Johnson Reprint Corporation.

Report of the Indian Immigrants Commission 1885-87. 1887. Pietermaritzburg: P. Davis & Sons.

Riesman, David. 1950. *The Lonely Crowd*. New Haven: Yale University Press.

———. 1952. *Faces in the Crowd*. New Haven: Yale University Press.

Rooney, James F. 1982-83. "The Influence of Informal Control Sources Upon Adolescent Alcohol Use and Problems." *American Journal of Drug and Alcohol Abuse* 9.

SACHED. 1985. *Working Women*. Johannesburg: Raven Press.

Samuelson, L. H. nd. *Some Zulu Customs*. London: Church Printing Co.

Schapera, I., and B. Farrington (eds.). 1933. *The Earl Cape Hottentots*. Cape Town: The Van Riebeeck Society.

Smart, R. G., et al. 1979. *Alcohol and Drug Use Among Ontario Students in 1979 and Changes from 1977: Preliminary Findings*. Sub-study No. 1070. Toronto: Addiction Research Foundations.

Smart, R. G., and Murray, G. F. 1981. "A Review of Trends in Alcohol and Cannabis Use Among Young People." *Bulletin on Narcotics* 33.

Smart R. G., and Others. 1980. *A Methodology for Student Drug Use Surveys*. No. 50. Geneva: World Health Organization.

Smith, Andrew. 1939. *The Diary of Dr. Andrew Smith (1834-36)*. Vol. I. Ed. Percival Kirby. Cape Town: The Van Riebeeck Society.

Snyman, C. R. 1974. *Misdade Betreffende Afhanklikheidsvormende Medisyne*. Durban: Butterworths.

Social Science Data Archives (SSDA). 1983. *Drug Use in Australia: A Directory of Survey Research Projects*. Canberra: Australian National University.

Stayt, Hugh A. 1931. *The Bavenda*. London: Oxford University Press.

Stow, George W. 1905. *The Native Races of South Africa*. London: Swan Sonnenschein.

Suggs, David N., and Brian M. du Toit. 1985. "Socialization and Sobriety: Alcohol Use Among Students in a Southern County." *Florida Journal of Anthropology* 10/1.

Swanson, D. M., A. P. Bratrude, and E. M. Brown. 1971. "Alcohol Abuse in a Population of Indian Children." *Diseases of the Nervous System* 31.

Ten Rhyne, Wilhelm. 1933. *A Short Account of the Cape of Good Hope and of the Hottentots who Inhabit that Region*. Cape Town: The Van Riebeeck Society.

Topper, M. D. 1974. "Drinking Patterns, Culture Change, Sociability and Navajo Adolescents." *Addictive Diseases* 1.

Tylor, Josiah. 1891. *Forty Years Among the Zulus*. Boston: Congregational Sunday School Publishing Society.

Ungerleider, J. Thomas, and Therese Andrysiak. 1984. "Changes in the Drug Scene: Drug Use Trends and Behavioral Patterns." *Journal of Drug Issues* 14.

Urzua, Florenzano R., E. Mantelli, U. Madrid, A. M. Martini, and M. E. Zalazar. 1982. "Patterns of Drug, Alcohol and Tobacco Use Among High School Students in Santiago, Chile." *Bulletin on Narcotics* 34.

Van der Burgh, C. 1975. *Drugs and South African Youth*. Human Sciences Research Council Report No. S-38. Pretoria.

Vodra, Joan, and James Garbarino. 1988. "Social Influences on Adolescent Behavior Problems." In *Social Networks of Children, Adolescents and College Students*. ed. Suzanne Salzinger, John Antrobus and Muriel Hammer. Hillsdale, New Jersey: Lawrence Erlbaum Associates.

Watt, J. M., and M. G. Breyer-Brandwijk. 1932. *The Medicinal and Poisonous Plants of Southern Africa*. Edinburgh: E. and S. Livingstone.

Wechsler, Henry, and Mary McFadden. 1976. "Sex Differences in Adolescent Alcohol and Drug Use." *Journal of Studies of Alcohol* 37.

Wechsler, Henry, and Denise Thum. 1973. "Teen-Age Drinking, Drug Use, and Social Correlates." *Quarterly Journal of Studies in Alcohol* 34.

Weibel, J. 1982. *American Indians, Urbanization and Alcohol: A Developing Urban Drinking Ethos*. Special Population Issues. The National Institute on Alcohol Abuse and Alcoholism.

Weibel-Orlando, Joan. 1984. "Substance Abuse Among American Indian Youth: A Continuing Crisis." *Journal of Drug Issues* 14.

Westphal, E. O. J. 1963. "The Linguistic Prehistory of Southern Africa: Bush, Kwadi, Hottentot and Bantu Linguistic Relationships." *Africa* 33.

_____. 1971. "The Click Languages of Southern and Eastern Africa." In *Current Trends in Linguistics: Linguistics in Sub-Saharan Africa* ed. Jack Berry and Joseph H. Greenberg. The Hague: Mouton.

Winick, Charles. 1965. "Marihuana Use by Young People." In *Drug Addiction in Youth* ed. Ernest Harms. London: Pergamon Press.

MONOGRAPHS IN INTERNATIONAL STUDIES

Africa Series

ISBN Prefix 0-89680-

36. Fadiman, Jeffrey A. *The Moment of Conquest: Meru, Kenya, 1907.* 1979. 70pp.
    081-4 $ 5.50*

37. Wright, Donald R. *Oral Traditions From The Gambia: Volume I, Mandinka Griots.* 1979. 176pp.
    083-0 $15.00*

38. Wright, Donald R. *Oral Traditions From The Gambia: Volume II, Family Elders.* 1980. 200pp.
    084-9 $15.00*

41. Lindfors, Bernth. *Mazungumzo: Interviews with East African Writers, Publishers, Editors, and Scholars.* 1981. 179pp.
    108-X $13.00*

43. Harik, Elsa M. and Donald G. Schilling. *The Politics of Education in Colonial Algeria and Kenya.* 1984. 102pp.
    117-9 $12.50*

44. Smith, Daniel R. *The Influence of the Fabian Colonial Bureau on the Independence Movement in Tanganyika.* 1985. x, 98pp.
    125-X $11.00*

45. Keto, C. Tsehloane. *American-South African Relations 1784-1980: Review and Select Bibliography.* 1985. 159pp.
    128-4 $11.00*

46. Burness, Don, and Mary-Lou Burness, ed. *Wanasema: Conversations with African Writers*. 1985. 95pp.
129-2 $11.00*

47. Switzer, Les. *Media and Dependency in South Africa: A Case Study of the Press and the Ciskei "Homeland"*. 1985. 80pp.
130-6 $10.00*

48. Heggoy, Alf Andrew. *The French Conquest of Algiers, 1830: An Algerian Oral Tradition*. 1986. 101pp.
131-4 $11.00*

49. Hart, Ursula Kingsmill. *Two Ladies of Colonial Algeria: The Lives and Times of Aurelie Picard and Isabelle Eberhardt*. 1987. 156pp.
143-8 $11.00*

50. Voeltz, Richard A. *German Colonialism and the South West Africa Company, 1894-1914*. 1988. 143pp.
146-2 $12.00*

51. Clayton, Anthony, and David Killingray. *Khaki and Blue: Military and Police in British Colonial Africa*. 1989. 235pp.
147-0 $18.00*

52. Northrup, David. *Beyond the Bend in the River: African Labor in Eastern Zaire, 1865-1940*. 1988. 195pp.
151-9 $15.00*

53. Makinde, M. Akin. *African Philosophy, Culture, and Traditional Medicine*. 1988. 175pp.
152-7 $13.00*

54. Parson, Jack, ed. *Succession to High Office in Botswana. Three Case Studies*. 1990. 443pp.
157-8 $20.00*

55. Burness, Don. *A Horse of White Clouds*. 1989. 193pp.
158-6 $12.00*

56. Staudinger, Paul. *In the Heart of the Hausa States.* Tr. by Johanna Moody. 1990. 2 vols. 653pp.
160-8 $35.00*

57. Sikainga, Ahmad Alawad. *The Western Bahr Al-Ghazal Under British Rule: 1898-1956.* 1991. 183pp.
161-6 $15.00*

58. Wilson, Louis E. *The Krobo People of Ghana to 1892: A Political and Social History.* 1991. 254pp.
164-0 $20.00*

59. du Toit, Brian M. *Cannabis, Alcohol, and the South African Student: Adolescent Drug Use 1974-1985.* 1991. 166pp.
166-7 $17.00*

Latin America Series

8. Clayton, Lawrence A. *Caulkers and Carpenters in a New World: The Shipyards of Colonial Guayaquil.* 1980. 189pp, illus.
103-9 $15.00*

9. Tata, Robert J. *Structural Changes in Puerto Rico's Economy: 1947-1976.* 1981. xiv, 104pp.
107-1 $12.00*

11. O'Shaughnessy, Laura N., and Louis H. Serra. *Church and Revolution in Nicaragua.* 1986. 118pp.
126-8 $12.00*

12. Wallace, Brian. *Ownership and Development: A Comparison of Domestic and Foreign Investment in Colombian Manufacturing.* 1987. 186pp.
145-4 $10.00*

13. Henderson, James D. *Conservative Thought in Latin America: The Ideas of Laureano Gomez.* 1988. 150pp.
148-9 $13.00*

14. Summ, G. Harvey, and Tom Kelly. *The Good Neighbors: America, Panama, and the 1977 Canal Treaties.* 1988. 135pp.
149-7 $13.00*

15. Peritore, Patrick. *Socialism, Communism, and Liberation Theology in Brazil: An Opinion Survey Using Q-Methodology.* 1990. 245pp.
156-X $15.00*

16. Alexander, Robert J. *Juscelino Kubitschek and the Development of Brazil.* 1991. 429pp.
163-2 $25.00*

17. Mijeski, Kenneth J., ed. *The Nicaraguan Constitution of 1987: English Translation and Commentary.* 1990. 355pp.
165-9 $25.00*

Southeast Asia Series

31. Nash, Manning. *Peasant Citizens: Politics, Religion, and Modernization in Kelantan, Malaysia.* 1974. 181pp.
018-0 $12.00*

38. Bailey, Conner. *Broker, Mediator, Patron, and Kinsman: An Historical Analysis of Key Leadership Roles in a Rural Malaysian District.* 1976. 79pp.
024-5 $ 8.00*

44. Collier, William L., et al. *Income, Employment and Food Systems in Javanese Coastal Villages.* 1977. 160pp.
031-8 $10.00*

45. Chew, Sock Foon and MacDougall, John A. *Forever Plural: The Perception and Practice of Inter-Communal Marriage in Singapore.* 1977. 61pp.
030-X $ 8.00*

47. Wessing, Robert. *Cosmology and Social Behavior in a West Javanese Settlement.* 1978. 200pp.
072-5 $12.00*

48. Willer, Thomas F., ed. *Southeast Asian References in the British Parliamentary Papers, 1801-1972/73: An Index.* 1978. 110pp.
033-4 $ 8.50*

49. Durrenberger, E. Paul. *Agricultural Production and Household Budgets in a Shan Peasant Village in Northwestern Thailand: A Quantitative Description.* 1978. 142pp.
071-7 $10.00*

50. Echauz, Robustiano. *Sketches of the Island of Negros.* 1978. 174pp.
070-9 $12.00*

51. Krannich, Ronald L. *Mayors and Managers in Thailand: The Struggle for Political Life in Administrative Settings.* 1978. 139pp.
073-3 $11.00*

56A. Duiker, William J. *Vietnam Since the Fall of Saigon.* Updated edition. 1989. 383pp.
162-4 $17.00*

59. Foster, Brian L. *Commerce and Ethnic Differences: The Case of the Mons in Thailand.* 1982. x, 93pp.
112-8 $10.00*

60. Frederick, William H., and John H. McGlynn. *Reflections on Rebellion: Stories from the Indonesian Upheavals of 1948 and 1965.* 1983. vi, 168pp.
111-X $ 9.00*

61. Cady, John F. *Contacts With Burma, 1935-1949: A Personal Account.* 1983. x, 117pp.
114-4 $ 9.00*

63. Carstens, Sharon, ed. *Cultural Identity in Northern Peninsular Malaysia.* 1986. 91pp.
116-0 $ 9.00*

64. Dardjowidjojo, Soenjono. *Vocabulary Building in Indonesian: An Advanced Reader.* 1984. xviii, 256pp.
118-7 $26.00*

65. Errington, J. Joseph. *Language and Social Change in Java: Linguistic Reflexes of Modernization in a Traditional Royal Polity.* 1985. xiv, 211pp.
120-9 $20.00*

66. Binh, Tran Tu. *The Red Earth: A Vietnamese Memoir of Life on a Colonial Rubber Plantation.* Tr. by John Spragens. Ed. by David Marr. 1985. xii, 98pp.
119-5 $11.00*

68. Syukri, Ibrahim. *History of the Malay Kingdom of Patani.* Tr. by Conner Bailey and John N. Miksic. 1985. xix, 113pp.
123-3 $12.00*

69. Keeler, Ward. *Javanese: A Cultural Approach.* 1984. xxxvi, 523pp.
121-7 $18.00*

70. Wilson, Constance M., and Lucien M. Hanks. *Burma-Thailand Frontier Over Sixteen Decades: Three Descriptive Documents.* 1985. x, 128pp.
124-1 $11.00*

71. Thomas, Lynn L., and Franz von Benda-Beckmann, eds. *Change and Continuity in Minangkabau: Local, Regional, and Historical Perspectives on West Sumatra.* 1986. 363pp.
127-6 $16.00*

72. Reid, Anthony, and Oki Akira, eds. *The Japanese Experience in Indonesia: Selected Memoirs of 1942-1945.* 1986. 411pp., 20 illus.
132-2 $20.00*

73. Smirenskaia, Zhanna D. *Peasants in Asia: Social Consciousness and Social Struggle.* Tr. by Michael J. Buckley. 1987. 248pp.
134-9 $14.00

74. McArthur, M.S.H. *Report on Brunei in 1904.* Ed. by A.V.M. Horton. 1987. 304pp.
135-7 $15.00

75. Lockard, Craig Alan. *From Kampung to City. A Social History of Kuching Malaysia 1820-1970.* 1987. 311pp.
136-5 $16.00*

76. McGinn, Richard. *Studies in Austronesian Linguistics.* 1988. 492pp.
137-3 $20.00*

77. Muego, Benjamin N. *Spectator Society: The Philippines Under Martial Rule.* 1988. 232pp.
138-1 $15.00*

78. Chew, Sock Foon. *Ethnicity and Nationality in Singapore.* 1987. 229pp.
139-X $12.50*

79. Walton, Susan Pratt. *Mode in Javanese Music.* 1987. 279pp.
144-6 $15.00*

80. Nguyen Anh Tuan. *South Vietnam Trial and Experience: A Challenge for Development.* 1987. 482pp.
141-1 $18.00*

81. Van der Veur, Paul W., ed. *Toward a Glorious Indonesia: Reminiscences and Observations of Dr. Soetomo.* 1987. 367pp.
142-X $16.00*

82. Spores, John C. *Running Amok: An Historical Inquiry.* 1988. 190pp.
140-3 $14.00*

83. Tan Malaka. *From Jail to Jail.* Tr. and ed. by Helen Jarvis. 1990. 3 vols. 1,226pp.
150-0 $55.00*

84. Devas, Nick. *Financing Local Government in Indonesia.* 1989. 344pp.
153-5 $16.00*

85. Suryadinata, Leo. *Military Ascendancy and Political Culture: A Study of Indonesia's Golkar.* 1989. 222pp.
179-9 $15.00*

86. Williams, Michael. *Communism, Religion, and Revolt in Banten.* 1990. 356pp.
155-1 $16.00*

87. Hudak, Thomas John. *The Indigenization of Pali Meters in Thai Poetry.* 1990. 237pp.
159-4 $15.00*

88. Lay, Ma Ma. *Not Out of Hate: A Novel of Burma.* Tr. by Margaret Aung-Thwin. Ed. by William Frederick. 1991. 222pp.
167-5 $20.00*

ORDERING INFORMATION

Orders for titles in the Monographs in International Studies series may be placed through the Ohio University Press, Scott Quadrangle, Athens, Ohio 45701-2979 or through any local bookstore. Individuals should remit payment by check, VISA, MasterCard, or American Express. People ordering from the United Kingdom, Continental Europe, the Middle East, and Africa should order through Academic and University Publishers Group, 1 Gower Street, London WC1E, England. Orders from the Pacific Region, Asia, Australia, and New Zealand should be sent to East-West Export Books, c/o the University of Hawaii Press, 2840 Kolowalu Street, Honolulu, Hawaii 96822, USA.

Other individuals ordering from outside of the U.S. should remit in U.S. funds to the Ohio University Press either by International Money Order or by a check drawn on a U.S. bank. Most out-of-print titles may be ordered from University Microfilms, Inc., 300 North Zeeb Road, Ann Arbor, Michigan 48106, USA.

Prices do not include shipping charges and are subject to change without notice.

8 cuios
last 2000
D/D 3/05